FACE
UP

FACE
UP

THE ESSENTIAL MAKE-UP HANDBOOK
RUBY HAMMER AND MILLIE KENDALL
WITH TAMARA STURTZ

EBURY
PRESS

FIRST PUBLISHED IN GREAT BRITAIN IN 2000

1 3 5 7 9 10 8 6 4 2

FIRST PUBLISHED BY EBURY PRESS

RANDOM HOUSE, 20 VAUXHALL BRIDGE ROAD, LONDON SW1V 2SA

RANDOM HOUSE AUSTRALIA (PTY) LIMITED

20 ALFRED STREET, MILSONS POINT, SYDNEY, NEW SOUTH WALES 2061, AUSTRALIA

RANDOM HOUSE NEW ZEALAND LIMITED

18 POLAND ROAD, GLENFIELD, AUCKLAND 10, NEW ZEALAND

RANDOM HOUSE SOUTH AFRICA (PTY) LIMITED

ENDULINI, 5A JUBILEE ROAD, PARKTOWN 2193, SOUTH AFRICA

THE RANDOM HOUSE GROUP LIMITED REG. NO. 954009

WWW.RANDOMHOUSE.CO.UK

A CIP CATALOGUE RECORD FOR THIS BOOK IS AVAILABLE FROM THE BRITISH LIBRARY.

MAKE-UP: RUBY HAMMER

PHOTOGRAPHY: STEVE HIETT
ART DIRECTION: STEVE HIETT
DESIGN: STEVE HIETT WITH EMERAUDE NICOLAS
GRAPHIC ASSISTANT: JULIE ATLAN
EDITOR: EMMA CALLERY
STYLING: TAMARA STURTZ
HAIR: FERNANDO TORRENT
DIGITAL IMAGING: CORE LONDON LTD

ISBN 0 09 187475 0

COLOUR ORIGINATION BY COLORLITO SRL, MILAN - ITALY
PRINTED AND BOUND IN SINGAPORE BY TIEN WAH PRESS

CONTENTS

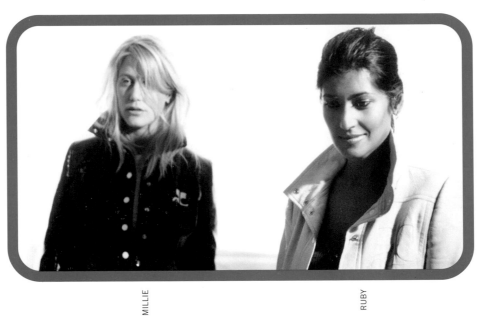

MILLIE

RUBY

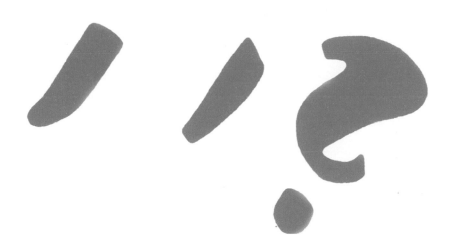

who are ruby and millie ?

I HAVE KNOWN MILLIE FOR TEN YEARS FROM WHEN SHE WAS MANAGING THE SHU UEMURA BOUTIQUE IN LONDON, AND RUBY EIGHT, WHEN WE WORKED TOGETHER ON PHOTOGRAPHIC SHOOTS FOR *MARIE CLAIRE* AND *HARPERS & QUEEN*. IN THAT TIME I HAVE GAINED SO MUCH, NOT ONLY IN LOYAL FRIENDSHIPS, BUT IN KNOWLEDGE TOO. WHEN RUBY & MILLIE GOT TOGETHER – MAKE-UP ARTIST AND BEAUTY VIRTUOSO – IT WAS A PARTNERSHIP THAT COULD ONLY GO FROM STRENGTH TO STRENGTH AND THEIR SUCCESS HAS BEEN BUILT ON DETERMINATION, ENTHUSIASM AND HARD WORK. AS TWO WORKING MOTHERS I DON'T KNOW HOW THEY FIND THE TIME TO ACHIEVE EVERYTHING THAT THEY DO. I CAN ONLY HAVE ADMIRATION AND RESPECT FOR THEIR DEDICATION.

WHEN LOOKING FOR QUOTES ON THE MAGAZINES I'VE WORKED ON, THEY ARE ALWAYS THE FIRST I WOULD CALL FOR THEIR WEALTH OF KNOWLEDGE AND BRILLIANT TIPS, SO IT MAKES SENSE THAT THIS KNOWLEDGE BE PUT DOWN IN A BOOK. AFTER ALL, MUCH OF THEIR PHILOSOPHY IS ABOUT SHARING THEIR KNOWLEDGE WITH AS MANY WOMEN AS POSSIBLE. THEY STRONGLY BELIEVE THAT GOOD COSMETICS AND GOOD ADVICE SHOULD BE AVAILABLE TO ABSOLUTELY EVERYBODY AND ANYBODY WHO WANTS TO KNOW.

SINCE WORKING WITH THEM ON THIS BOOK I HAVE LEARNT SO MUCH. I NOW ACTUALLY KNOW HOW TO APPLY MY MAKE-UP PROPERLY, AND IT MAKES ALL THE DIFFERENCE. I KNOW HOW TO MAKE MY EYES STAND OUT, MY BLUSHER LAST ALL NIGHT INSTEAD OF HALF AN HOUR, AND WHEN I GET SPOTS ON MY CHIN I KNOW THAT WEARING RED LIPSTICK REALLY DOES DRAW ATTENTION AWAY FROM THEM. ADMITTEDLY, I'VE HAD TO ADD A FEW MORE PRODUCTS TO MY MAKE-UP BAG, BUT I'VE THROWN A FEW OUT TOO, LIKE THE MASCARA I'D HAD FOR A YEAR AND THE FUCHSIA PINK LIPSTICK I ONLY USED ONCE. I LOOK AT MY FACE PROPERLY IN THE MORNINGS AND, AS MILLIE TOLD ME WOULD HAPPEN, I'VE STARTED TO LIKE IT MORE. I NOW HAVE THE SKILLS TO MAKE THE MOST OF WHAT I'VE GOT AND IT HAS GIVEN ME THAT EXTRA BOOST OF CONFIDENCE. AND I'VE STARTED TO EXPERIMENT. I MIGHT START THE DAY WITH PINK GLOSS ON MY LIPS, CHANGE TO RED AFTER LUNCH AND END IT WITH PLUM LIPSTICK. BUT MOST OF ALL I ENJOY IT AND I'M HAVING FUN. LOTS OF IT.

TAMARA STURTZ

ruby & millie – the philosophy

RUBY & MILLIE HAVE CREATED A UNIQUE AND FRESH APPROACH TO BEAUTY, RECOGNIZING THE NEEDS OF THE INDIVIDUAL OVER STRUCTURED TECHNIQUE AND THE IMPORTANCE OF BUILDING CONFIDENCE. IT IS A PHILOSOPHY THAT REACHES, AND CAN BE INTERPRETED BY, ALL WOMEN, REGARDLESS OF AGE, COLOUR OR LIFESTYLE. BOTH RUBY AND MILLIE ARE IN THEIR THIRTIES, BUT THEY HAVE BEEN TEENAGERS, THEY'VE BEEN IN THEIR TWENTIES, THEY HAVE MOTHERS, GRANDMOTHERS, AUNTS, COLLEAGUES AND FRIENDS. THEY ARE CONSTANTLY DEALING WITH PEOPLE WITH DIFFERENT CONCERNS THAT MAY NOT BE PERSONAL TO THEM, AND BECAUSE OF THIS THEY ARE VERY AWARE OF WHAT WOMEN WANT OUT THERE.

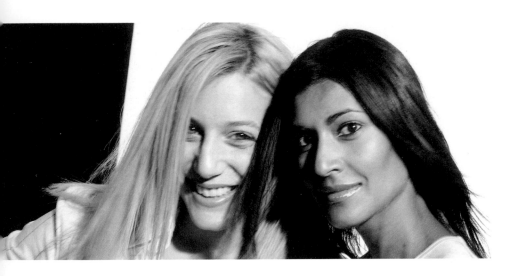

THEY UNDERSTAND THE IMPORTANCE OF HAVING PRODUCTS THAT PERFORM BOTH SIMPLY, EFFECTIVELY AND CAN BE RELIED ON, BUT ARE ALSO FUN AND ACCESSIBLE. THEY ARE BOTH WORKING MOTHERS WITH EXTRAORDINARILY BUSY LIVES WHO WANT TO LOOK THEIR BEST AND SO ATTEMPT TO MAKE LIFE SIMPLE, ORGANIZED AND PRACTICAL SO IT CAN RUN AS SMOOTHLY AS POSSIBLE.

ONE OF THE BRILLIANT THINGS ABOUT THEIR PARTNERSHIP IS THAT IT IS A POOLING OF RESOURCES, KNOWLEDGE AND EXPERIENCE. WHEN MILLIE FIRST MET RUBY SHE HAD NEVER THOUGHT OF PUTTING ON CONCEALER AFTER HER FOUNDATION, BUT SHE LEARNT SOMETHING THAT SHE NOW LIVES BY AND THAT MAKES HER LOOK BETTER. RUBY IS A MAKE-UP ARTIST AND THAT'S HER PROFESSION BUT SHE IS THE FIRST TO ADMIT THAT IT DOESN'T MAKE HER THE WORLD EXPERT ON EVERY FORM OF MAKE-UP. SHE WATCHES MILLIE PUT THINGS TOGETHER, USE A COLOUR A CERTAIN WAY, WHICH HAS NOTHING TO DO WITH BEING PROFESSIONAL OR NOT, AND SHE THINKS 'WOW'. IT INSPIRES HER.

A BIG PART OF THEIR PHILOSOPHY IS THAT EVEN THOUGH 'RUBY & MILLIE' COMES FROM TWO INDIVIDUALS, THEY ARE OPEN TO MYRIAD INFLUENCES, FROM THEIR PEERS, FRIENDS, JOURNALISTS, MODELS, MAKE-UP ARTISTS AND OTHER GREAT WOMEN OUT THERE. THEY WANT MAKE-UP TO BE PERFECT, BUT THEY ALSO KNOW THAT IT HAS TO BE REALISTIC AND ACHIEVABLE. NO ONE IS PERFECT. AND BECAUSE THEY USE THEMSELVES IN ALL THEIR ADVERTISING AND PROMOTIONAL PICTURES, WHEN WOMEN COME TO THEIR COUNTER FOR ADVICE, RUBY & MILLIE UNDERSTAND THAT THEY'RE COMING TO REAL WOMEN.

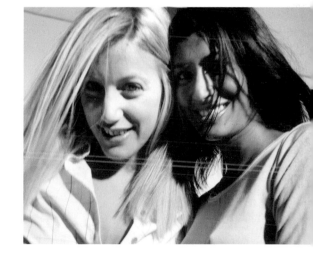

THE RUBY & MILLIE PHILOSOPHY IS ABOUT GAINING CONFIDENCE THROUGH THE MEDIUM OF MAKE-UP. BECAUSE ALL WOMEN ARE DIFFERENT, IT IS BASED AROUND THE ASSESSMENT OF YOUR OWN FACE SO THAT YOU NOT ONLY DEVELOP A MORE POSITIVE APPROACH TO YOURSELF BUT GAIN CONFIDENCE IN USING MAKE-UP. JUST LIKE A NEW PAIR OF SHOES OR THE PERFECT HAIRCUT, COSMETICS ARE SPECIAL IN THEIR ABILITY TO MAKE US FEEL BETTER ABOUT OURSELVES. MAKE-UP SHOULDN'T BE A MASK TO HIDE BEHIND, BUT YOU CAN USE IT TO DISGUISE FLAWS AND ENHANCE YOUR GOOD BITS WITH A MERE STROKE OF COLOUR.

face up

THIS BOOK IS NOT ABOUT RIGID RULES AND INSTRUCTIONS. IT ADDRESSES THE 'WHY' OF MAKE-UP BEFORE THE 'HOW'. IT'S ABOUT THINKING FOR YOURSELF AND ABANDONING THE RULES RATHER THAN FOLLOWING THEM. IT IS SIMPLE, LOGICAL AND MAKES SENSE, YET ALLOWS FOR INTERPRETATION AND, MOST OF ALL, INSPIRATION. BY BREAKING THE 'STEP-BY-STEP' MOULD FOLLOWED BY THE CURRENT CROP OF BEAUTY BOOKS, THIS BOOK SETS ITSELF APART, OFFERING WOMEN A UNIQUE AND ORIGINAL PHILOSOPHY THAT THEY CAN APPLY TO THEMSELVES. IT RECOGNIZES THAT MODERN WOMEN NO LONGER FEEL THE

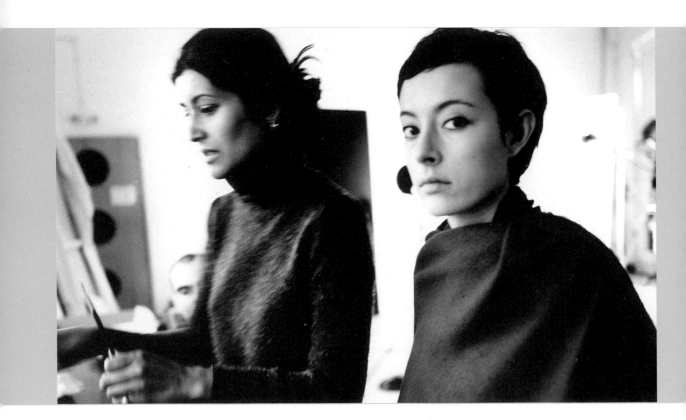

NEED TO FOLLOW THE PACK BUT WANT THE RIGHT TO EXPRESS THEMSELVES AS INDIVIDUALS. RUBY & MILLIE APPRECIATE THAT PERSONALITY AND SELF-CONFIDENCE CREATES INDIVIDUAL BEAUTY AND THIS IS ENHANCED BY THE ABILITY TO ASSESS YOUR OWN MAKE-UP NEEDS. THE AIM OF THIS BOOK IS TO SIMPLY DEFINE WHAT IS ACHIEVABLE AND TO REINFORCE THAT ANYTHING IS ACCEPTABLE.

IF YOU WANT TO STAND ON YOUR HEAD TO PUT ON YOUR EYELINER, AND IT WORKS FOR YOU, THAT'S OKAY. THERE ARE NO RULES. THERE ARE TIPS AND TECHNIQUES THAT CAN BE USED TO SIMPLIFY AND ADDRESS CERTAIN ISSUES, BUT EVERYTHING IS ACCEPTABLE.

RUBY & MILLIE BELIEVE THAT THERE ARE TOO MANY WOMEN OUT THERE WHO ARE EITHER AFRAID OF MAKE-UP OR SEE IT AS A FRIVOLOUS BUY. THIS NEEDS TO CHANGE. MAKE-UP HAS BEEN A PART OF OUR SOCIETY FOR HUNDREDS OF YEARS AND IT SPEAKS ALL KINDS OF LANGUAGES. APART FROM ANYTHING ELSE, IT'S A WAY OF EXPRESSING OURSELVES. BUT MOST IMPORTANTLY, IT'S ABOUT EXPERIMENTING WITH MAKE-UP, ENJOYING IT AND HAVING LOTS AND LOTS OF FUN.

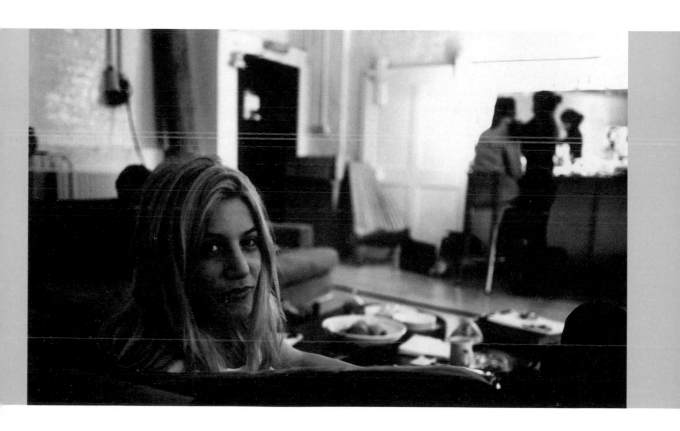

chapter 1

LOOKING GOOD IS ABOUT SELF-CONFIDENCE: KNOWING WHO YOU ARE, WORKING WITH WHAT YOU'VE GOT AND ACCEPTING YOUR FEATURES. WE'RE VERY LUCKY THAT WE ALL HAVE DIFFERENT FACES AND DIFFERENT FEATURES, THEY MAKE US UNIQUE AND INDIVIDUAL. AND WE CAN PLAY UP WHAT WE LIKE AND PLAY DOWN WHAT WE DON'T.

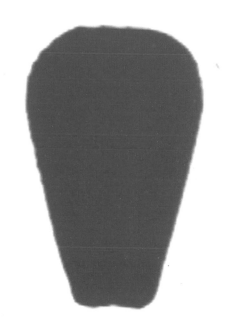

the real you

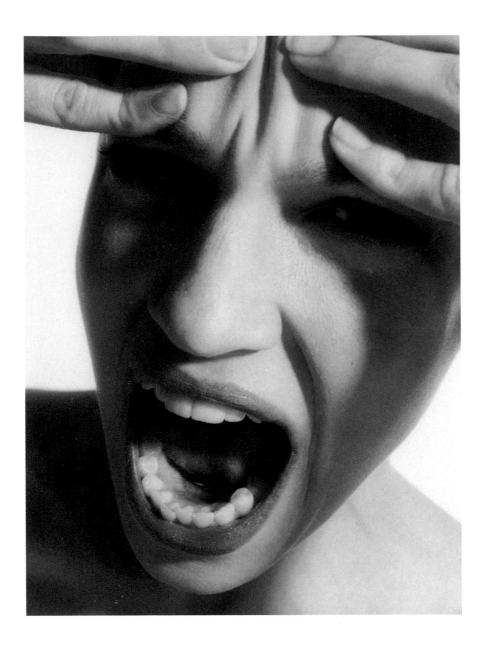

assessing
make-up

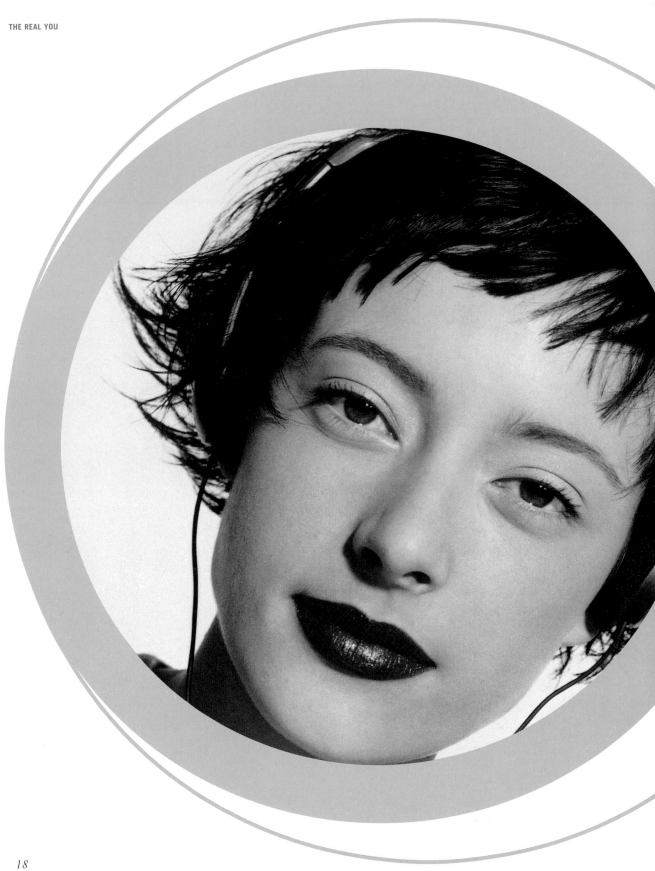

Don't create an unrealistic ideal before you have even started, because the chances are, you'll never achieve it. Be honest with yourself. Our tip is to sit or stand in front of a mirror with clean skin and really examine your face. Turn your head around and look at it from all angles. Are your eyes bright, are your eyelashes nice and thick, what shape are your lips? But remember that nobody scrutinizes your face as closely as you do.

If you're concerned about how other people look at you and assess you when you first meet them, remember that at least 80 per cent of those people you meet will not be looking at your appearance, but at who you are as a person. If you walk into a room with an air of confidence, people are going to think that you look a lot better than if you creep in looking apologetic.

Second, assess your lifestyle. Do you have to get up and go to work every morning, are you a mother at home or a mixture of the two? Decide what you want to achieve from your appearance. Do you want to be seen as someone who is confident and in control of her business or demure yet sexually exciting, or maybe you don't really care either way. Then ask yourself how much time you have. There's no point in deciding on a look that's going to take half an hour to put on when you only have ten minutes every morning.

Third, know your limitations. Know that you can alter your appearance with make-up but only to a certain degree. You can probably alter it more by coming across with the right attitude. For example, if you want to

appear very sexy but you don't have the confidence to wear a push-up bra and a low-cut top, then know that is your limitation. In the same way, vampy red lipstick and black eyeliner is not going to change the way you are. Millie knows that she is never going to be tall and thin, so she works with clothes and make-up that make the most of her curvaceous figure and bubbly personality. Work your make-up around who you are.

Also aim to accept what you've got. When Ruby was sixteen she was paranoid about stretch marks, but as she's got older, they're the least of her worries. She'd rather improve other bits about her, as a person. It doesn't mean that she doesn't look at her skin and wish it was better, but she now has the confidence to think, 'Well this is what I've been given, and apart from surgery, what is realistically achievable?' Make peace with what you've got and then you'll enjoy what you have.

● Experiment with make-up. It's not like getting a haircut where you're stuck with it for the next few months.

● You can do it in the privacy of your own home – a bit of peace and quiet, your favourite music, a glass of wine – and have a go.

● Look at it and see if you like it. Ask yourself, 'Could I walk out of the door like this?' If you don't like it, all you have to do is wipe it off.

● Get to know your features and how they all tie in together. The more you experiment, the more you'll know what suits you.

● And don't worry about being vain, it's not taboo to look at yourself in the mirror.

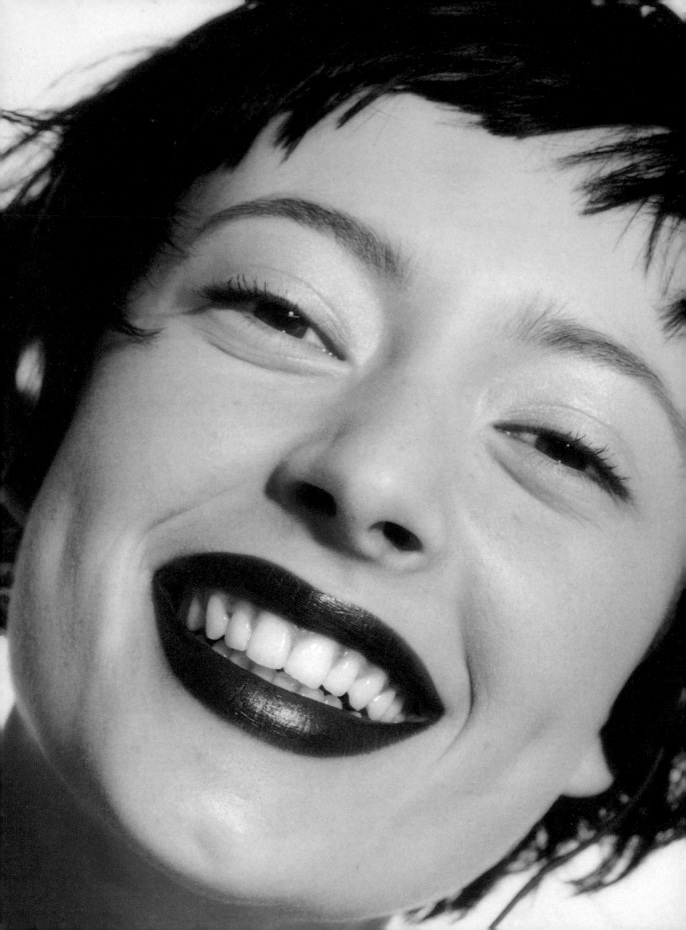

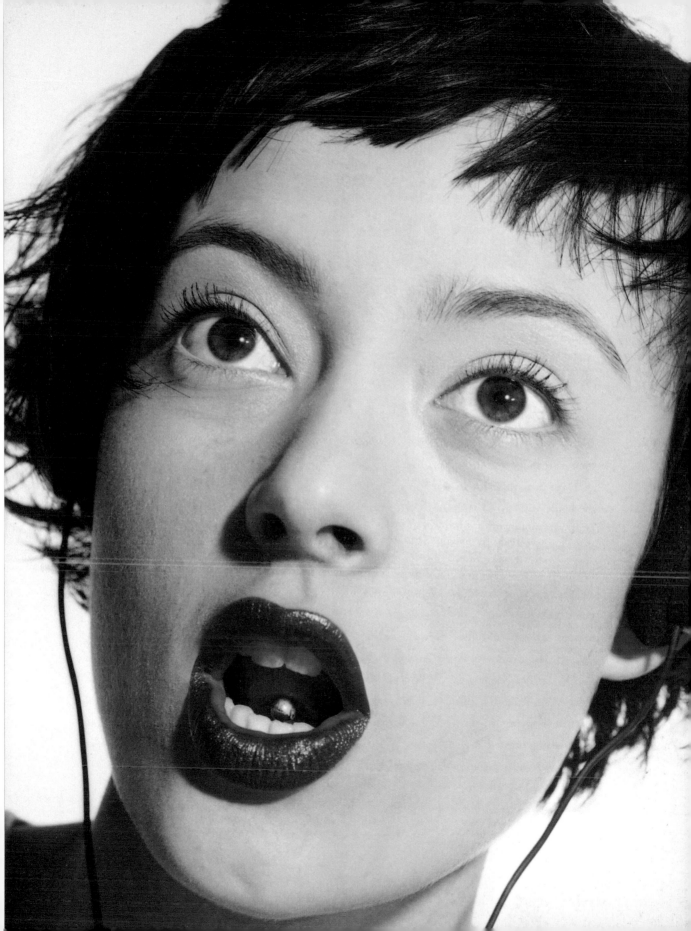

When you see a make-up artist working in the studio, she always uses a mirror to prepare the model. Eyes are deceptive. How you feel about a person is going to make them beautiful or ugly in your eyes. But the mirror never lies. The mirror gives you some distance so you can be more objective:

● Close up, you may think you've blended a colour on to your face perfectly, but when you stand back you can properly judge what you've done and see what it really looks like.

● For example, when you look in the mirror you might notice that your eyebrows don't match. When Millie looks at Ruby she can't tell that one of Ruby's eyebrows is higher than the other. But when she looks at her in the mirror she can see it, because the mirror defines what is going on.

● It is also helpful to have a side mirror because people also look at you from both sides as well as the back, and either up or down, depending on your height.

● Millie uses her side mirror when applying concealer because she can see where she needs it around the bridge of her nose better than if she were looking at it straight on.

Once you start looking at yourself in the mirror more, you'll probably find that you start liking yourself more. You'll start to appreciate your features and it can be a great confidence builder. So often the assumption is that if you scrutinize your face, you'll find all the things that are wrong. But turn this on its head and say, if you're not looking, how are you going to find all those good things about you?

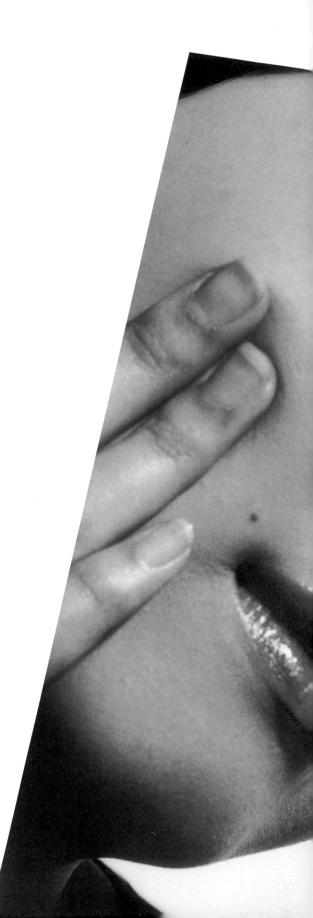

MIRROR MIRROR

great expectation

Once you've become comfortable with looking at yourself in the mirror, address your expectations and what you're going to do, today. Ask yourself what the mirror is reflecting.

● How do I enhance this or what can I do to make that look better?

● What is achievable and what isn't?

● Are you going to be a mother today, a business woman, are you having lunch with a friend, going on a date or going out after work?

Irrespective of whether you use a lot of make-up or not, know how to use it or don't, love it or hate it, most of us, whatever our age, have a few products lying around, whether it's an over-stuffed make-up bag or the odd lipstick at the bottom of our handbag. And usually there is some kind of self-imposed ritual in which these products are applied, all with a quick glance in the mirror. Now is the time to break down that ritual. Instead of going through the motions, ask yourself if you really need that concealer , or is it time to update that blusher?

If a colour doesn't work on your lips, it doesn't mean that it won't look great on your cheeks, eyes or nails, but the only way you will know this is by experimenting.

Ruby is often asked does she always know from start to finish what she's going to do when she's making up a face? The answer is no. When working on a model, she looks at the face first and determines the end result she wants to achieve. Is it a soft, gleaming, fresh face, or something strong and dramatic? Is it dewy, powdered or matte? Once she has a picture in her head, Ruby then picks out the products needed to achieve that.

The condition of your skin may even determine what you do, but you won't know until you've looked at it closely. The best way to break it down is in the order of our chapters:

● skin

● base

● face

● and colour.

It's logical. Look at your skin and decide what you're going to clean it with, then look at your face, do you want concealer, foundation, powder, or a combination of just two? Look at the rest of your face, do you need blusher today, have you got peeky skin, do you want contours, a little bit of shimmer or do you want to look matte? And then go on to colour: lipstick, eye shadow, nails. It's really very logical.

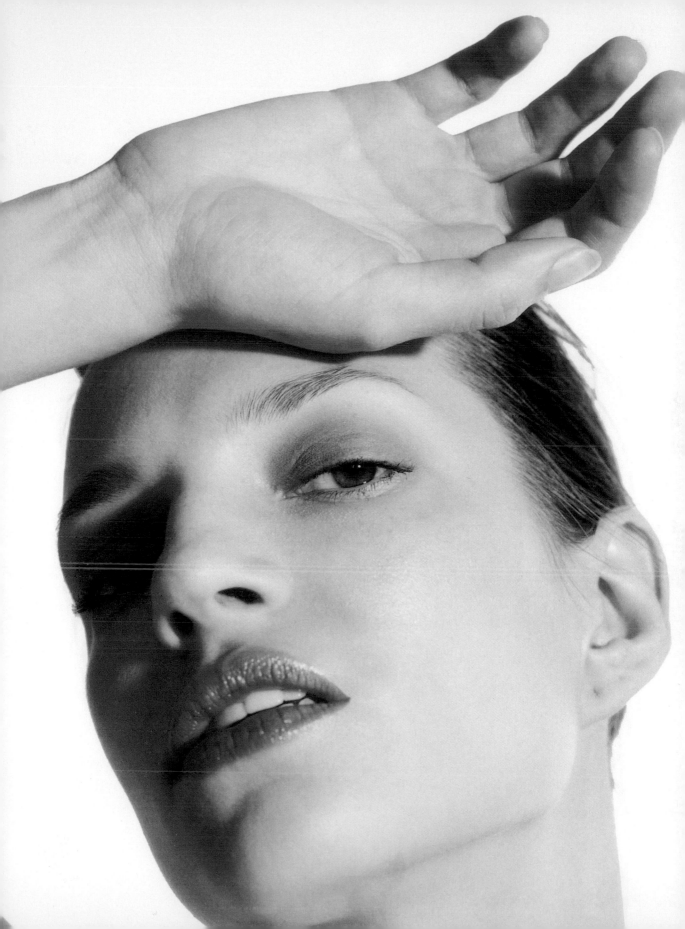

chapter 2

CLEAN, HEALTHY, RADIANT SKIN. ISN'T THAT WHAT WE ALL WANT? WE CAN'T CHANGE WHAT WE WERE BORN WITH, BUT WE CAN DEFINITELY MAKE THE MOST OF WHAT WE'VE GOT.

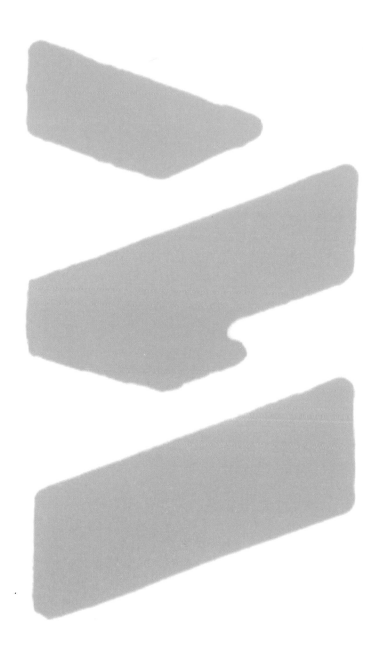

skin win

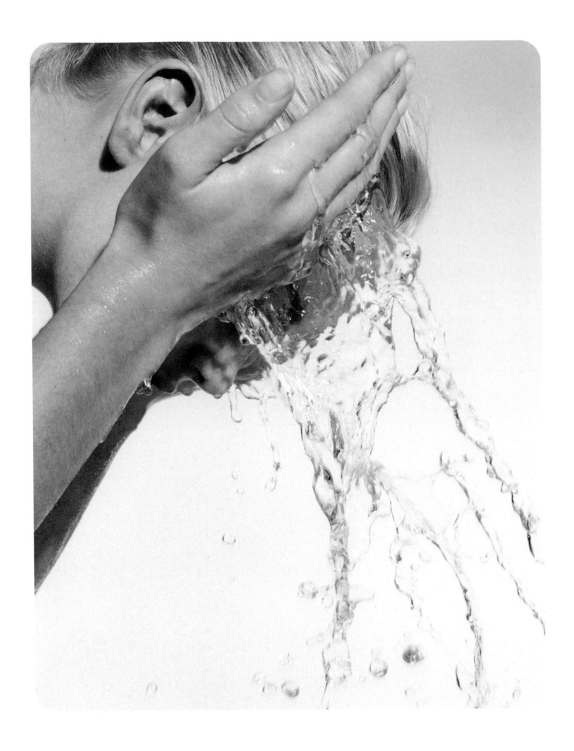

preparation

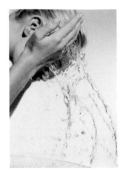

'ENJOY YOUR REGIME, IT'S NOT MEANT TO BE A CHORE. TREAT YOURSELF TO AN EXPENSIVE CREAM ONCE IN A WHILE. WE'RE NOT SAYING YOU SHOULD SPEND LOADS OF TIME IN THE BATHROOM, JUST SPEND IT DIFFERENTLY.'

Skin care is about preparation. Make-up is going on to your face, so you must start off with the best skin possible. If it's greasy it will swallow up all your make-up, yet if it's too dry, it will start to separate and flake around your nose. Sound familiar? If your skin is clean and moist, your make-up will look its best. Begin by looking at yourself in the mirror. And really look. We're assuming you have a pretty good skin care regime, we're not here to tell you how to do it. We just want you to get the most out of your skin. There are six key things to look at:

- your genes, and you're stuck with those.
- sun protection – it's never too late to start.
- your skin care regime, by now you will know whether your skin is oily, dry, prone to spots, whatever.
- smoking.
- the environment, such as central heating, wind, rain, and cold weather.
- your general health and whether you're exercising and flushing out the toxins.

Cleanse and nourish is the key. But first of all, assess your skin. Do you feel as well as you did yesterday, did you have a late night, have you got your period, have you got a spot coming up, or do you look more radiant than you have in ages? When you wake up, instead of wandering into the bathroom and going through the motions with your eyes shut, look at your face and feel it. Does it feel dry or rough anywhere, is it slightly more oily than normal? Feel under the chin, look round your nose, look at the pores. Is there anything different from yesterday or last week? And if there is, what are you going to do about it?

Have a selection of products on hand – one milk and one oil cleanser perhaps, a toner, a light moisturizer, a richer one for dry days, something for zapping spots, that miracle lift product for when you haven't had enough sleep. And there will be some days when you feel a splash of water and a light moisturizer is all that you need.

cleanse ...

There are tons of cleansers around – gel, foam, cream, milk, soap, oil – but remember that a cleanser is exactly that. It's for cleaning the face and not a problem solver as such so it's important to choose the right one for you. When you cleanse, remember you are washing your face, and will probably deplete your skin of some of its natural moisture whatever product you use. You then replace it with your toner and moisturizer.

The idea is to cleanse in a gentle way that removes everything from your face. If you feel clean afterwards and your skin feels a little tight, you've done it. What type of cleanser you choose is up to you. Millie loves oil-based ones because dirt adheres to oil much better. Cream cleansers are more diluted but good for when you don't need such a deep cleanse. Ruby prefers a cream cleanser but doesn't feel comfortable taking it off with cotton wool. It absorbs the product and doesn't absorb the dirt properly. Instead she uses a hot flannel. If you want to use cotton wool, wet it first and the product will sit on the surface instead of being absorbed into it.

The first thing Ruby does when she cleanses her face, is wash her hands. This is very important. She then rubs the cleanser in her hands to warm it up, and starting from the bottom of her neck, she works her way up in circular motions, concentrating on problem areas such as around the nose, chin and forehead, for a good 30 seconds. She then removes the cleanser and dirt with her hot flannel, leaving the skin feeling clean and bright. After cleansing, Millie splashes with warm water followed by cold. Be careful that the water isn't too hot or too cold as this can burst the capillaries on your face. And don't forget to clean your neck and behind your ears, they're part of your face too. Even if you have not been wearing any make-up, you need to cleanse every day to get rid of environmental dirt and pollutants.

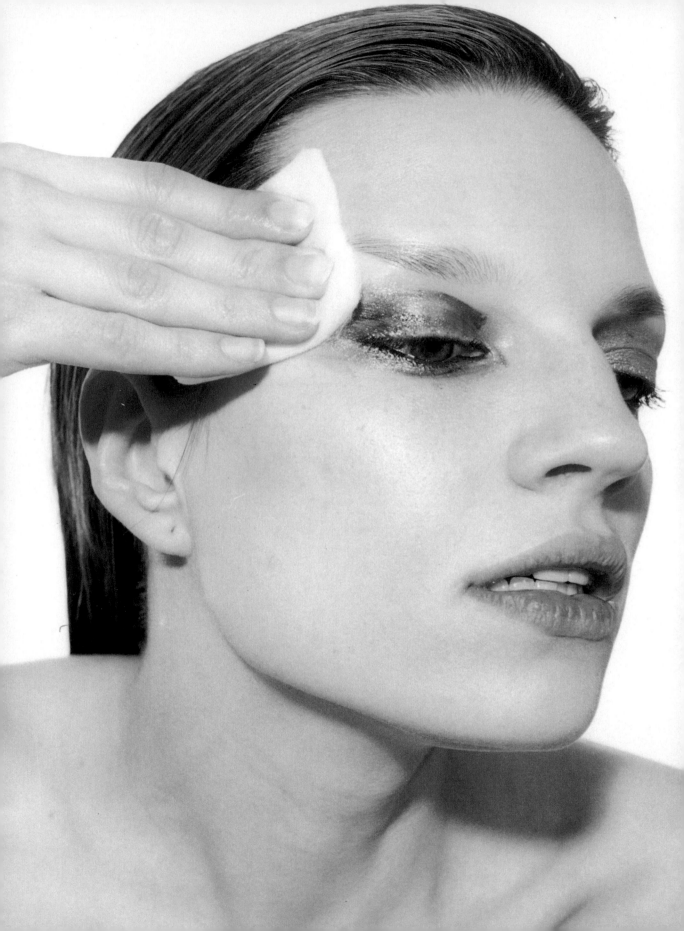

REMOVING EYE MAKE-UP

■ BEFORE YOU CLEANSE YOU MUST REMOVE YOUR EYE MAKE-UP. THIS OUGHT TO BE YOUR FIRST STEP IN YOUR CLEANSING REGIME BECAUSE IT IS SUCH A FRAGILE AREA. MILLIE TENDS TO USE THE SAME CLEANSER ON HER EYES AS SHE DOES FOR HER FACE, BUT THIS WORKS BECAUSE IT'S AN OIL CLEANSER AND SHE JUST USES IT MORE GENTLY. USING A Q-TIP DIPPED IN CLEANSER, SHE ROLLS IT DOWN HER LASHES TO REMOVE THE MASCARA, RUBS IT GENTLY UNDER THE EYE TO WIPE OFF ANY EYELINER AND SMEARS IT OVER HER EYELID.

■ HAVING LOOSENED THIS MAKE-UP, SHE THEN GOES ON TO CLEANSE THE REST OF HER FACE.

■ TAKE INTO ACCOUNT HOW MUCH EYE MAKE-UP YOU HAVE ON AND WHAT TYPE IT IS. IF YOU ARE WEARING WATERPROOF MASCARA, HEAVY EYELINER OR SOMETHING GLITTER-BASED, YOU ARE GOING TO HAVE TO DO A PRETTY THOROUGH JOB WHEN REMOVING IT AND YOU WILL PROBABLY NEED A SPECIFIC EYE MAKE-UP REMOVER.

■ IF YOU HAVE ON SOMETHING VERY LIGHT, THEN YOUR NORMAL CLEANSER WILL PROBABLY DO, BUT REMEMBER THAT IT WON'T GET RID OF WATERPROOF MAKE-UP. USE A DAMP COTTON PAD OR A Q-TIP LIKE MILLIE, AND HOLD IT OVER THE EYE FOR 30 SECONDS. THIS AVOIDS ANY RUBBING, SCRAPING OR PULLING AND ALLOWS THE EYE MAKE-UP TO BREAK DOWN AND DISSOLVE. GENTLY WIPE AWAY ONCE OR TWICE.

■ NEVER USE TOILET PAPER TO REMOVE EYE MAKE-UP, IT'S TOO HARSH AND IS A BIG NO NO.

tone ...

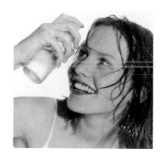

Toner has not been very fashionable of late, but skin needs water (moisture), and toner helps replace it. There is also no doubt that it feels good as it is refreshing and revitalizing. What kind of toner you use is up to you. They used to be astringent and skin-stripping, but most toners now are very mild and contain very little if no alcohol. You don't necessarily need to use it all the time, and at other times you may just want to use a toner on its own when you know you have cleansed very well the night before.

Toner also closes the pores after cleansing, preparing the skin for moisturizing. If you are not using a spray toner, gently pat it on to the skin with a moistened cotton pad to give your skin that wonderful massage effect.

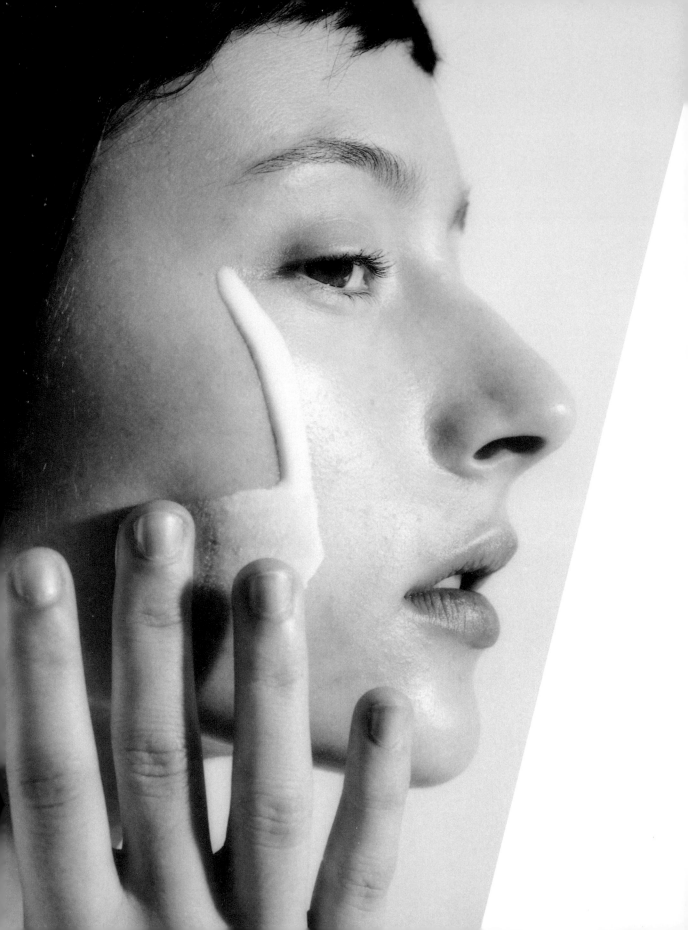

'IF YOU PUT MAKE-UP ON TO DIRTY SKIN IT DOESN'T FEEL NICE, AND IT WILL STICK IN FUNNY PLACES IF YOUR SKIN ISN'T WELL NOURISHED. APART FROM PREPARING THE SKIN FOR MAKE-UP, THIS THREE-STEP PROCESS GIVES YOU THE SAME EFFECT AS A FACIAL MASSAGE. YOU'RE TOUCHING YOUR FACE WITH YOUR FINGERS AND IT'S VERY PAMPERING. YOU'RE ALSO ENCOURAGING THE BLOOD TO THE SURFACE OF THE SKIN WHICH WILL GET YOU LOOKING RADIANT.'

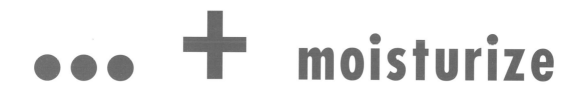

... + moisturize

There is no denying the comfort your skin feels after you've applied a moisturizer, whether it's a thick cream or a thin lotion. It feels nice and you can feel the effect immediately. It locks in moisture and lubricates the skin, giving you a smooth surface, allowing your make-up to go on more easily. Moisturizer also makes your skin supple, and most importantly it protects it. Always use a moisturizer, but you probably don't need to use it all over your face. A lot of us either use too little or too much. Look at where you need it, and don't forget your cheeks and forehead. Keep the changes in the seasons in mind – in the summer you may want something light and refreshing but with added sun protection, whereas in the winter you might need a richer cream to protect against the wind, cold and extra dryness.

We both believe that the cheaper brands are just as great as the more expensive ones. But in the end, it comes down to what works for you and what you can afford. An expensive cream may feel more luxurious, smell nicer and be of slightly better quality, but a cheaper brand will still protect and moisturize perfectly well.

chapter 3

CREATE THE PERFECT CANVAS FOR YOUR COLOUR WITH PRIMER, FOUNDATION,

CONCEALER AND POWDER. WHETHER IT'S A SHEER DEWY FINISH OR SOMETHING

COMPLETELY MATTE, YOUR BASE IS THE FIRST STEP IN ACHIEVING BEAUTIFUL MAKE-UP.

touching
base

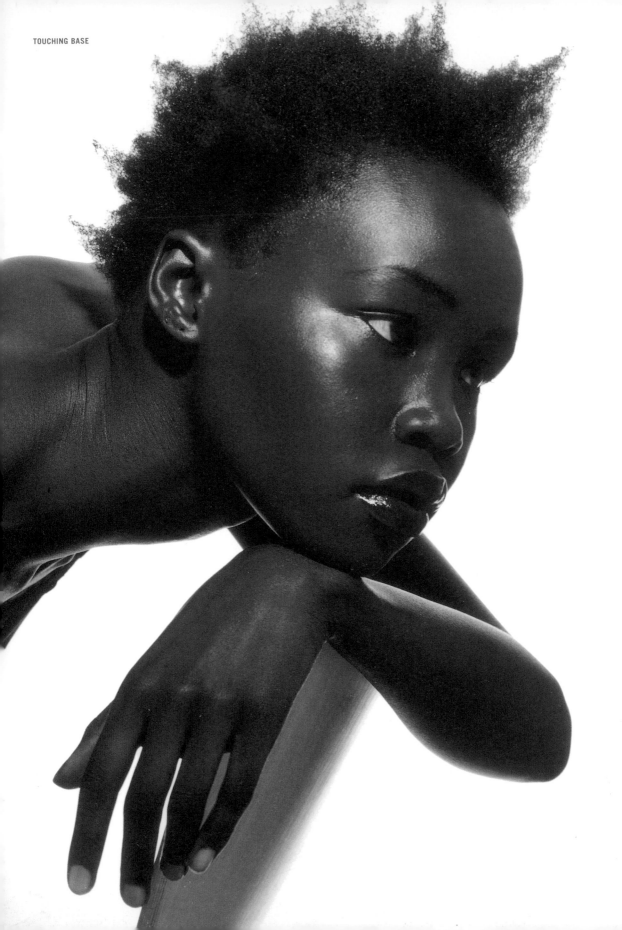

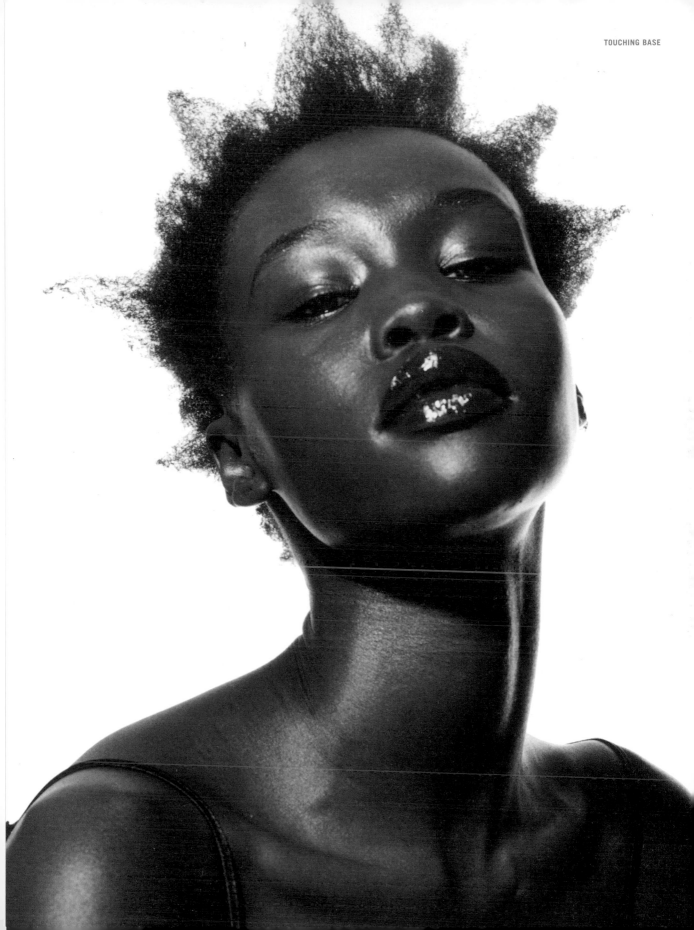

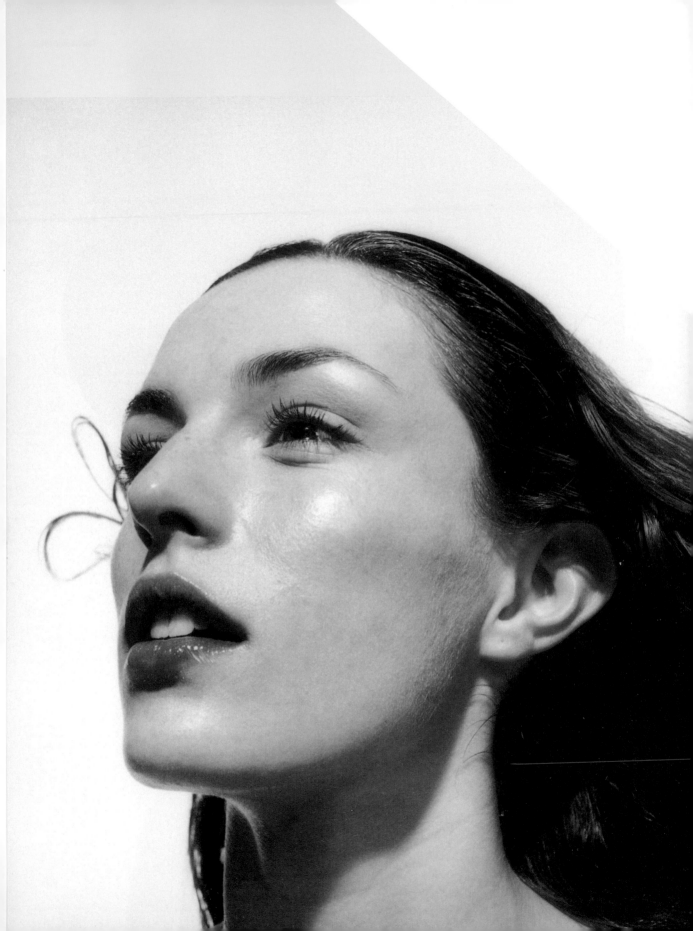

Once you've cleansed, toned and moisturized, you need to prepare your face for putting on colour. For many of us, moisturizing is the final stage of priming, but let us tell you about an additional step. Primer, or under-base as it is sometimes known, is our secret miracle product, and once you've tried it you probably won't want to do without it. There are four reasons why primer is so brilliant:

● The best surface to apply foundation to is a matte one, not all foundations go on smoothly to a well-moisturized or slightly oily skin.

● Once primer is applied your make-up will last a lot longer.

● Primer will heighten the effect of your foundation. Some are more liquid than others, enabling your foundation to look more dewy, some are shot with pearl so your make-up will be more light-catching, and others make your skin super matte so no shine will come through at all.

● Primer also prevents your make-up from sinking into the skin, and stops your natural oils from altering your make-up.

Millie is a great fan because it evens out her skin tone and helps smooth out any discoloration before she applies her base. She also suggests that if you don't want to wear any foundation, a bit of primer is a great product to use instead. It protects the skin and makes it look even without adding colour or coverage.

Because primer is relatively new to a lot of us, it's very easy to use too much, making it sit on the skin. As a result, anything else you put on over the top looks heavy. Start with a tiny pea-size – you can always add more – and, using a sponge, apply the primer to the larger areas of the face (cheeks and forehead) first and then blend it over the chin and nose. Just remember that less is more, but when used correctly it's a must-have for all make-up bags.

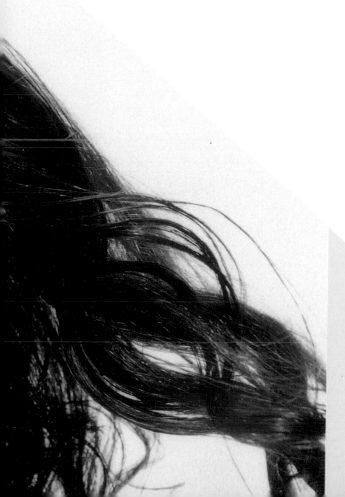

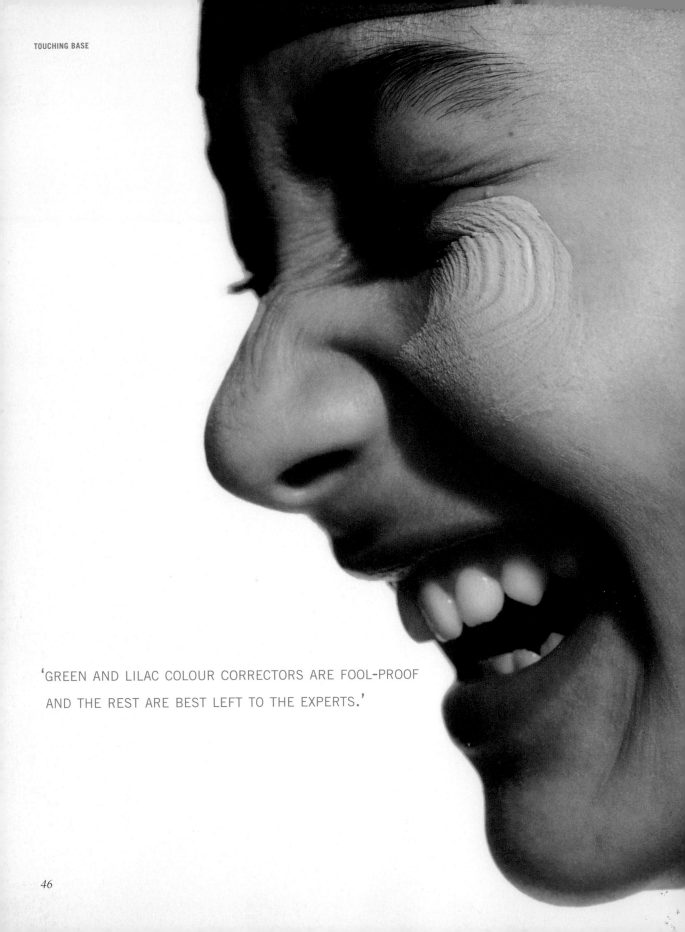

'GREEN AND LILAC COLOUR CORRECTORS ARE FOOL-PROOF
AND THE REST ARE BEST LEFT TO THE EXPERTS.'

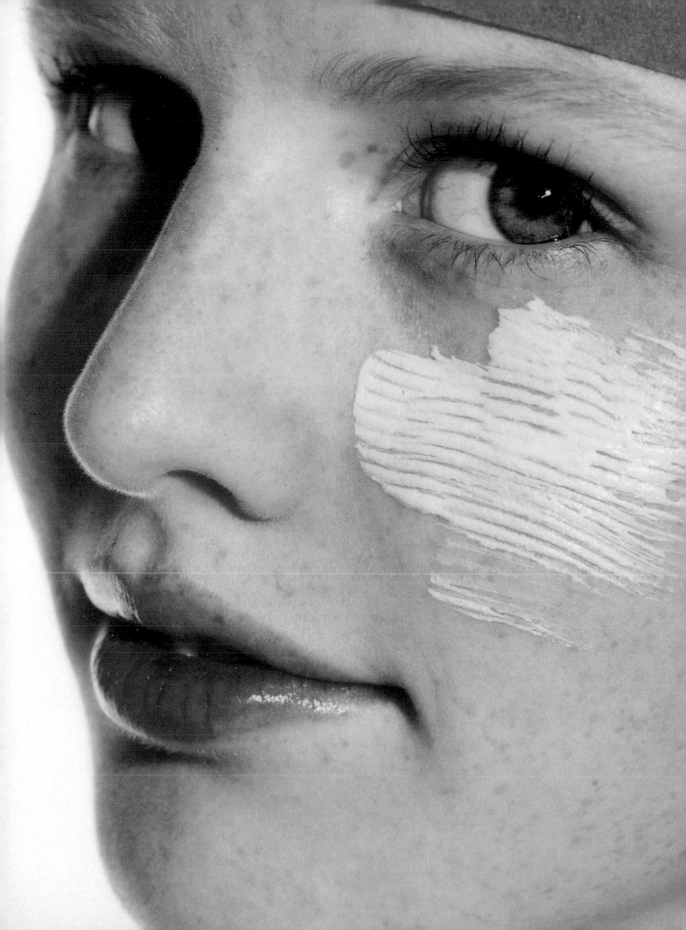

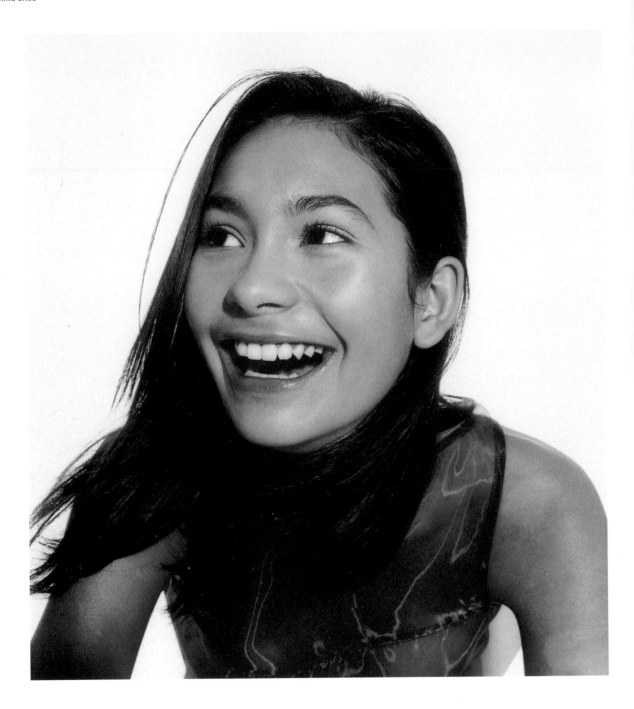

'WHAT YOU'RE TRYING TO ACHIEVE WITH FOUNDATION IS GOOD SKIN TONE THAT IS SMOOTH AND POLISHED LOOKING.'

colour correcting

So what exactly is a colour corrector? Just what it says, a colour liquid or cream that corrects the skin tone if necessary. It cosmetically allows you to put on a healthy vibrant face, where the alternative might be to have a facial.

The two most common colours are pale lilac, which reduces yellow in the skin, and a minty green, which tones down redness. Use either after your moisturizer and primer but before your base, or mixed into your foundation. If your primer isn't tinted — some

are, to even out colour — use a colour corrector instead. As with primer, use a little to start with and add more if you need to. You will probably only need a teeny bit here and there.

The brilliant thing about colour correctors is that they allow you to alter your base from day to day depending on what colour your skin is. As well as lilac and green there are other colours such as white, which can be used to tone down the colour of your base, and then there's black, blue, and the list goes on.

foundation

There are hundreds of foundations on the market — tinted moisturizer, fluid, cream, mousse, pancake, soufflé, stick, cream-to-powder — with almost as many finishes from velvet and dewy to matte and pearl. Decide on what finish you want to achieve. The colour will depend on how pale or dark your skin is, the coverage on how good your

skin is, and finish — matte, dewy, pearl — on personal choice. You might want a thicker foundation because you're looking a bit spotty but that doesn't mean you necessarily want it matte. Fortunately, with technology the way it is these days, you should be able to achieve that. However, you must be prepared to try before you buy.

APPLYING FOUNDATION

■ USE WHATEVER METHOD YOU LIKE – YOUR FINGERS, SPONGES IN ALL SHAPES AND SIZES, AND BRUSHES. APPLYING WITH YOUR FINGERS IS USER-FRIENDLY AND DOESN'T REQUIRE MUCH TECHNIQUE. A SPONGE OR BRUSH GIVES YOU MORE CONTROL. YOU CAN DISPERSE THE PRODUCT MORE EVENLY AND SMOOTHLY, AND IT'S MORE HYGIENIC.

■ WHAT YOU HAVE TO REMEMBER WHEN YOU'RE COVERING SUCH A HUGE AREA OF YOUR FACE, IS THAT IT'S NOT A FLAT SURFACE. IT HAS BLOOD VESSELS, HEAT, CONTOURS, MUSCLES, NOOKS AND CRANNIES, AND YOU NEED TO PICK A TOOL THAT CAN DEAL WITH ALL THESE AREAS.

■ EXPERIMENT WITH BOTH YOUR FINGERS AND A SPONGE, OR USE A BRUSH AROUND THE NOSE. RUBY USES A SPONGE TO APPLY HER BASE BUT ALWAYS FINE-TUNES IT WITH HER FINGERS TO MAKE IT LOOK MORE NATURAL.

■ NORMALLY THE LARGEST AREA TO CONCENTRATE ON IS THE CHEEK AREA. APPLY YOUR FOUNDATION TO THE CHEEKS FIRST AND THEN BLEND THE EXCESS ON TO AND DOWN THE T-ZONE.

■ IF YOU PUT A LOT OF FOUNDATION ON YOUR NOSE IT WILL LOOK LIKE YOU HAVE LOTS OF FOUNDATION ON YOUR NOSE. BECAUSE THE PORES ARE LARGER, THE PRODUCT SINKS INTO THEM AND BECOMES VERY OBVIOUS. REMEMBER, IT'S THE ONE AREA THAT REALLY STICKS OUT TOO.

■ BUILD UP LOTS OF THIN LAYERS INSTEAD OF ONE THICK ONE, AND ONLY APPLY THE FOUNDATION WHERE YOU NEED IT. IF YOU COVER THE WHOLE FACE FROM TOP TO BOTTOM, YOU'LL BE FLATTENING THE SURFACE, WHICH CAN LOOK MASK-LIKE AND LIFELESS.

■ SHE KNOWS IT CAN BE DIFFICULT, BUT MILLIE STRESSES THE IMPORTANCE OF WORKING FAST AS FOUNDATION DRIES VERY QUICKLY. SHE WORKS IN QUICK MOTIONS, PATTING AND BLENDING WITH A SPONGE OR HER FINGERS.

■ RUBY ALSO PATS ON HER FOUNDATION – PATTING IS DABBING AND CONTROLLING WHERE YOUR BASE GOES. IF YOU RUB, ALL YOU ARE DOING IS SPREADING THE FOUNDATION FROM ONE AREA TO ANOTHER.'

■ ALSO, BLEND IN ONE DIRECTION ONLY. WE ALL HAVE DOWNY FACIAL HAIR (OBVIOUS OR NOT), AND IF IT ALL LIES ONE WAY IT WILL GIVE THE ILLUSION OF A SMOOTHER FINISH.

■ A FINAL TIP FROM RUBY: ALWAYS START WITH LESS AND BUILD UP. YOU CAN ALWAYS ADD MORE.

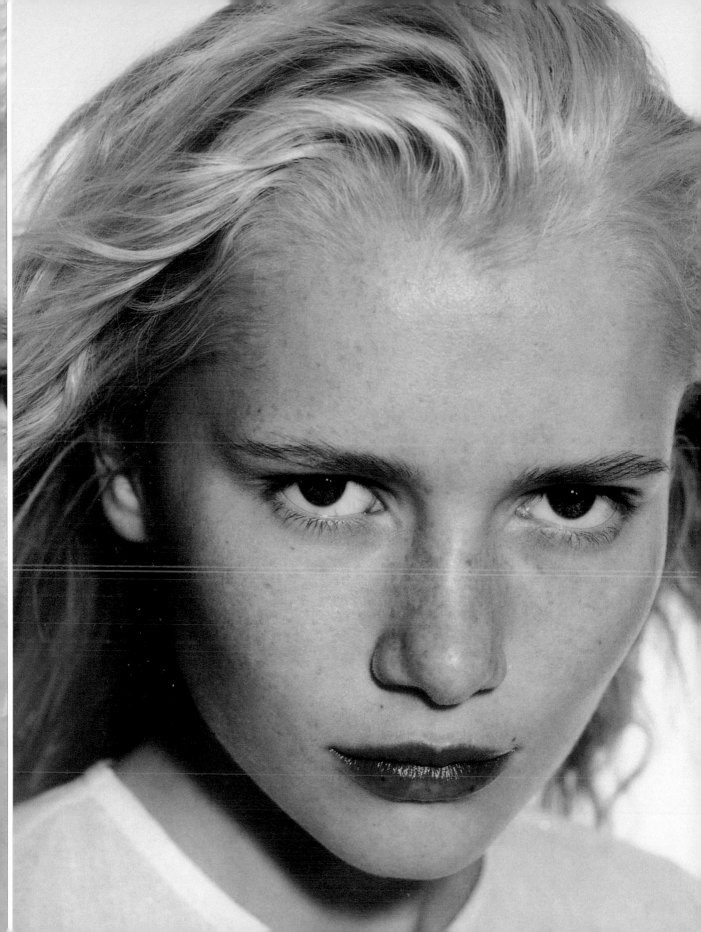

POW

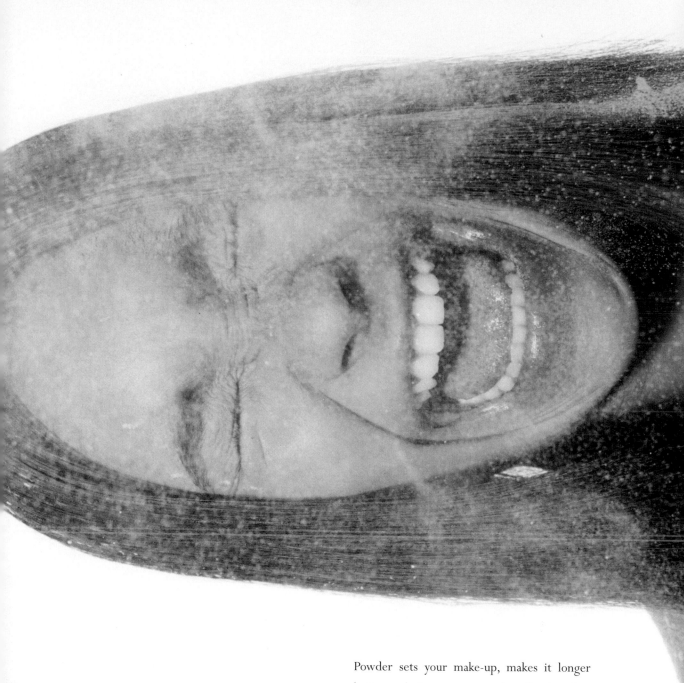

Powder sets your make-up, makes it longer
lasting and gives you a smooth, refined surface
for your colour to go on to. However, if you
have any other cream products to apply, cream
blusher for example, do that before you apply
your powder. The golden rule: powder on top
of powder and cream on top of cream.

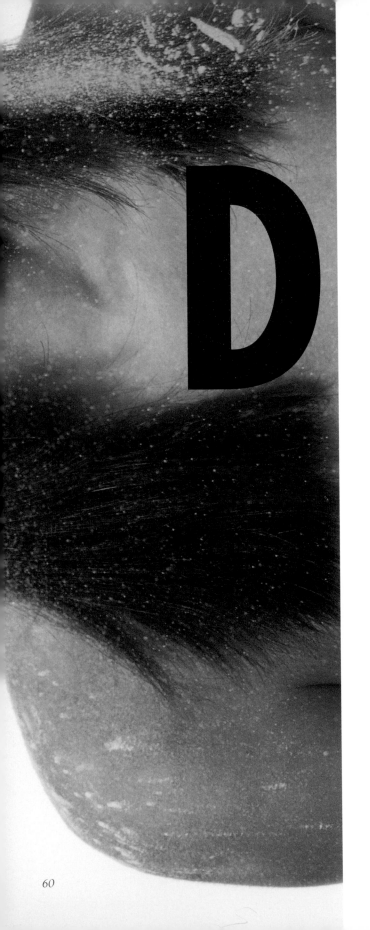

DER

There are two kinds of powder, loose and pressed. Loose is what you use to set your base, and pressed – which is basically loose powder with oil that has been pressed until it's compact – can be used on its own, on top of your primer or for touching up during the day. Don't use to set your foundation as the oil in both products will make the finished look too heavy. Millie suggests you keep loose powder at home and a pressed compact for carrying around.

Loose powder on top of foundation does not necessarily mean you're going to have a matte looking face. Today, powders are refined and sheer. Forget the old-fashioned talc formulations that your grandmother used to wear. As Ruby says, there is no reason to look like a 'baker's assistant'. Once you have set it on to your base it is absorbed, so what you end up with is the base again. If the powder is sitting on top of your skin, you've applied too much.

APPLYING POWDER

■ POWDERS COME IN ALL SHADES BUT THE MOST COMMON AND FOOLPROOF IS TRANSLUCENT, OR COLOURLESS, WHICH CAN BE WORN BY ALL SKIN COLOURS.

■ TO TEST THAT YOUR POWDER IS TRULY TRANSLUCENT, RUB THE POWDER INTO THE BACK OF YOUR HAND. IF IT DISAPPEARS, IT'S TRANSLUCENT. IF IT LEAVES A CHALKY RESIDUE, EITHER BIN IT OR DON'T BUY IT.

■ IF YOU WANT A COLOURED ONE, AGAIN MATCH IT TO YOUR SKIN COLOUR OR GO SLIGHTLY LIGHTER. NEVER GO DARKER AS IT CAN ALTER THE SHADE OF YOUR FOUNDATION. WITH TRANSLUCENT YOU CAN'T GO WRONG.

■ WHEN APPLYING POWDER YOUR CHOICE OF TOOLS ARE COTTON WOOL, A POWDER PUFF OR POWDER BRUSH. WE BOTH PREFER A PUFF BECAUSE IT GETS A MORE EVEN COVERAGE. USE A PUFF TO PRESS AND ROLL THE POWDER ON TO THE SKIN.

■ A BRUSH IS DOMED AND WON'T COVER ALL AREAS, BUT BECAUSE IT ONLY SKIMS THE SURFACE IT IS USEFUL TO SWEEP AWAY ANY EXCESS LEFT BY THE PUFF. KEEP THIS TECHNIQUE IN MIND, ESPECIALLY IF YOU'RE WEARING BLACK.

IF THE POWDER IS APPLIED WITH A BRUSH YOU'LL END UP WITH IT ALL OVER YOUR SHOULDERS LOOKING LIKE DANDRUFF. NO THANKS.

■ LIKE WITH FOUNDATION AND CONCEALER, BUILD UP YOUR POWDER IN LAYERS. AFTER FIVE OR TEN MINUTES (ALLOWING FOR THE POWDER TO SINK INTO THE SKIN), RUBY SUGGESTS APPLYING A THIN LAYER OF PRESSED POWDER AND YOU SHOULD FIND THAT IT WON'T BUDGE. THIS IS A GREAT TIP FOR WEDDINGS OR DAYS WHEN YOU NEED YOUR MAKE-UP TO LAST FOR HOURS.

■ THE SAME RULE GOES FOR BRONZING POWDER. APPLY IT AFTER YOU HAVE SET YOUR FOUNDATION WITH LOOSE POWDER.

■ BRONZING POWDER SHOULD ONLY GO ON SPECIFIC PARTS OF THE FACE – THE CHIN, CHEEKS, NOSE AND FOREHEAD. THESE ARE THE AREAS THAT STICK OUT AND ARE NORMALLY HIT BY THE SUN.

■ GO FOR SHADES OF POWDER WITH ONLY A HINT OF SHIMMER AS TOO MUCH SPARKLE WILL HAVE YOU LOOKING WORRYINGLY LIKE A DISCO BALL.

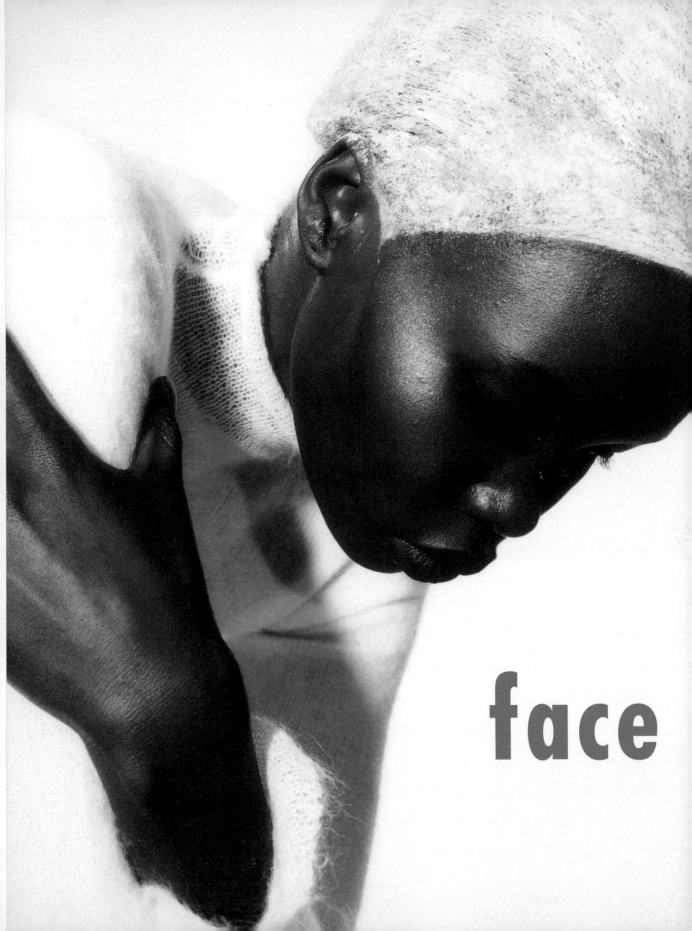

face

up

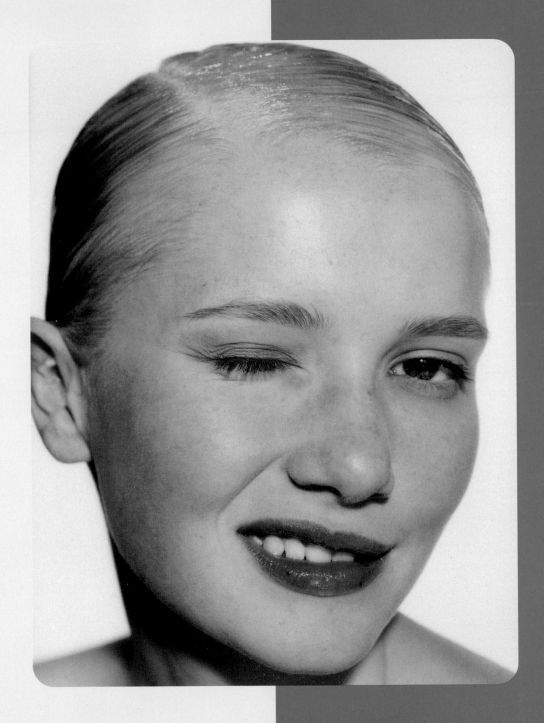

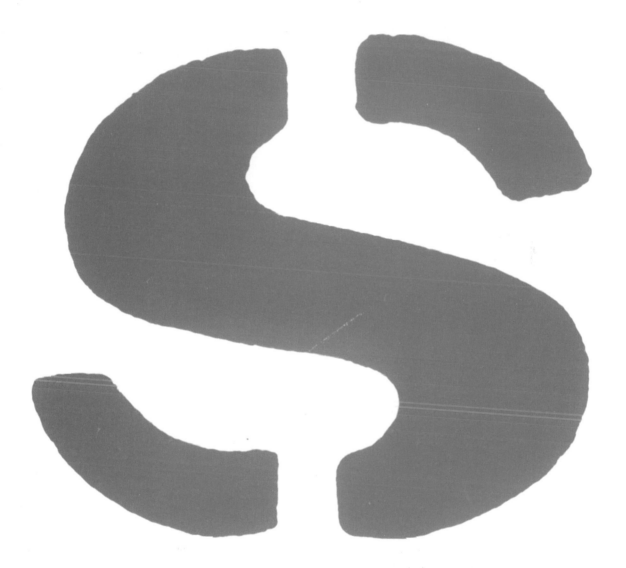

symmetry

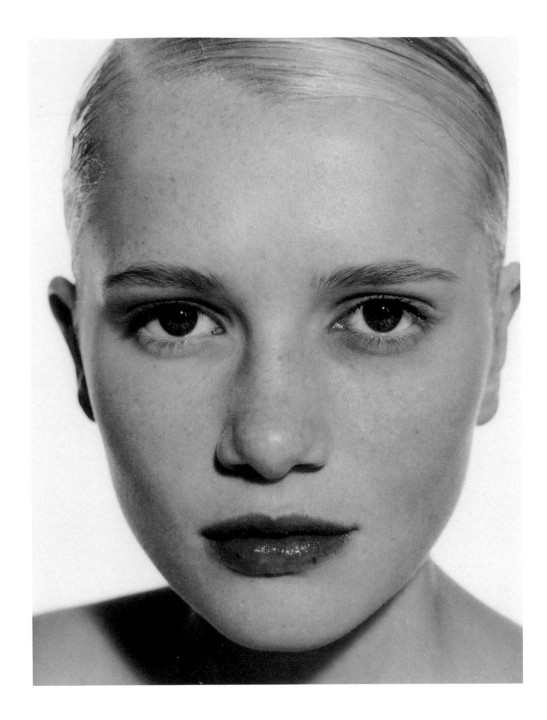

The first thing to remember is that nobody has a symmetrical face. If you photographed two left sides of your face and put them together they would look ridiculous. When applying make-up you have to take into account that each side of your face is different. If you did exactly the same make-up on both sides, the same shape eyebrows on both the left and right, for example, it's not going to look natural. Look at both sides individually and work to bring them together rather then match them up. With make-up, the aim is to make the face as even as possible, but not in an artificial and monochromatic way. It might be a matter of putting colour on the eyebrows and lengthening one slightly to balance them. Balance it as best as you can, but as naturally as you can.

Millie feels that this chapter is particularly important because she finds that when it comes to the actual face – eyebrows, contour, highlight and cheeks – it is generally overlooked, but it is the root of what a make-up artist does. And it's something we can all do. We can all learn to apply make-up but what we must learn to do is look, assess and think about what we're going to do.

'IT COMES DOWN TO KNOWING YOUR FACE, IT'S NOT GOING TO CHANGE DRASTICALLY OVER YOUR LIFETIME. LIKE WITH CLOTHES, YOU MAY WANT TO FOLLOW THE TRENDS BUT YOU WOULDN'T WEAR SOMETHING THAT DIDN'T SUIT YOU JUST FOR THE SAKE OF FASHION. THE SAME GOES FOR MAKE-UP.'

face shape

Everybody has a different face shape, and within that we have different features. Traditionally, we have been told there are four basic face shapes: oval, square, heart-shaped and round, with the ideal being oval. This was to be achieved with complex make-up techniques and contouring and highlighting. Forget it, it's dated and far too complicated. Everybody is individual, someone can have all their features in supposedly the wrong place and yet they are stunning and beautiful. When you look at your face, look at the individual features and ask yourself:

● Does it look imbalanced?

● Are your eyes big or small?

● Have you got a big nose, have you got thin lips or are they nice and full?

● Have you got a big forehead?

● Or have you got a really pointed chin?

You can do something about most of these things, albeit on a small scale, and there are little make-up tricks that can help you to do that. It's not like surgery, but it will help mask and put the attention on to something else.

And there are lots of ways of doing it. Millie suggests, for example, that if you have a wide jaw, instead of shading along the jaw bone to make it look narrower, which is dated and old-fashioned, increase the length of your eyebrows because it gives the illusion that the eye area is wider, therefore making the jaw line appear narrower. But Ruby says to keep in mind that these are marginal techniques. Don't think of it as a magic wand, they're great techniques but not life changing.

It might be that you don't have prominent cheekbones and that the trend is to wear cheek colour on the apple of your cheeks. Millie has small cheekbones, so this would make her face look wider. So she applies the cheek colour underneath the cheekbone area to look as though she has more cheek. But just because you think something doesn't suit you, don't just disregard it. If cream blushers are in and applied on the apple of your cheek, you can use that new texture, but as Millie says, because you know that you have hardly any cheekbones, you can just apply it 2cm (¾in) lower.

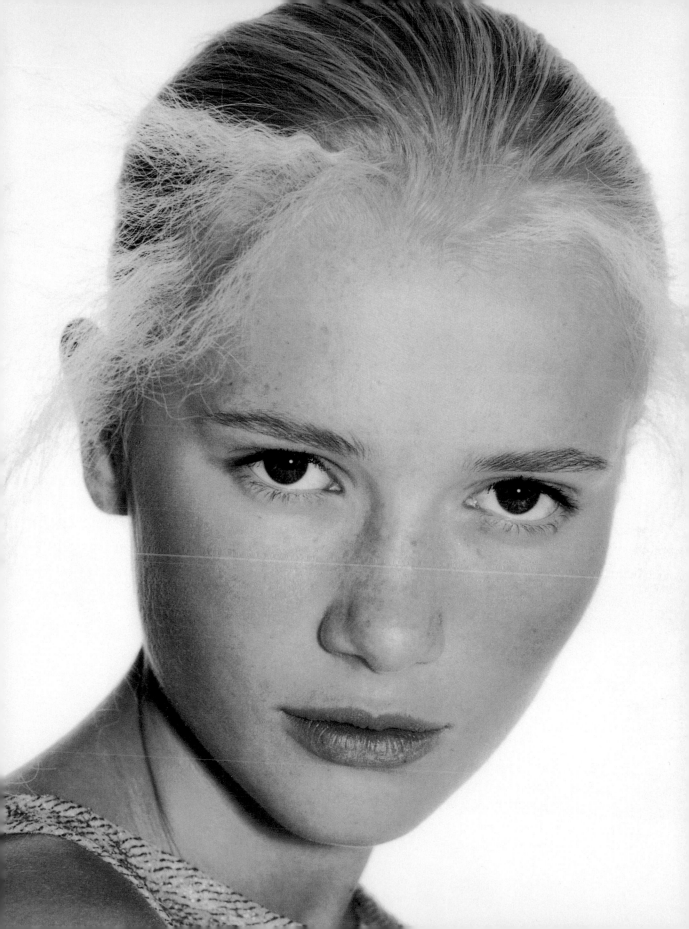

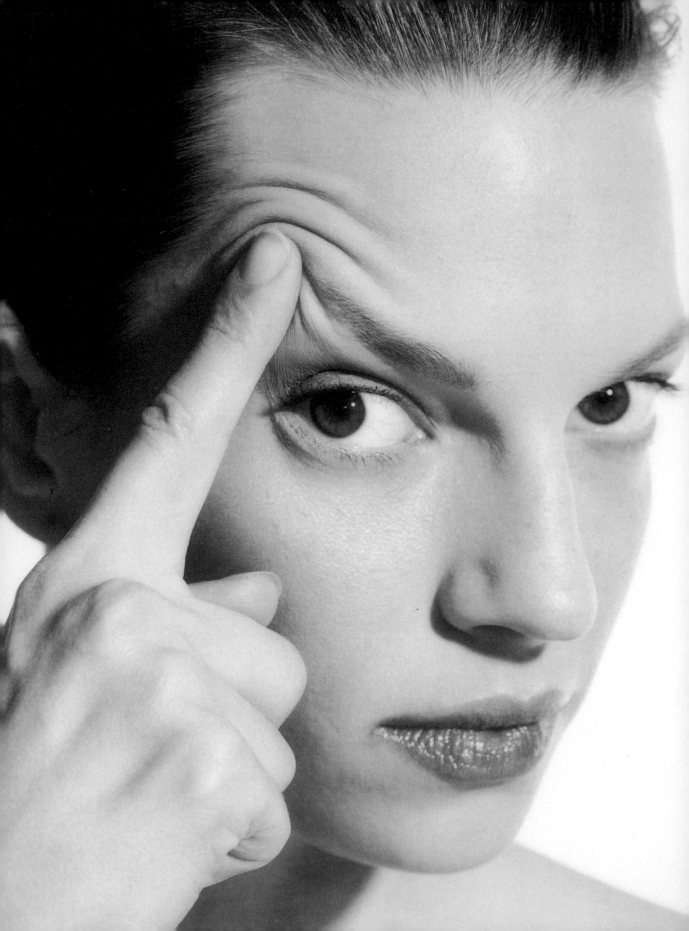

Eyebrows are the frame to your face. They give you expression and because of this they're very important. You can shape them, powder them, pluck them, shorten them, lengthen them, or you might not want to do anything other than brush them up and leave them. Whether she spends loads of time on them or not, Ruby never leaves her eyebrows all knitted and growing on top of one another. They are always brushed up so that they keep an open and clear expression.

The more you brush your brows up and pluck from underneath, the more space you're giving your eyelids for applying eye shadow. Getting your eyebrows into the right condition and shape not only gives your face a whole frame but it gives your eyes a frame too.

Before you apply any cosmetic to your eyebrows, assess the shape. Find the size and shape that suits you. Some women look better with thinner brows, and others with thicker. Assess your natural hair growth. Like with the hair on your head, what you were born with probably looks best if it's just groomed. Unless the damage has already been done, don't completely eradicate them and start again, because it's unlikely that you can achieve a better look than the one you were born with.

eyebrows

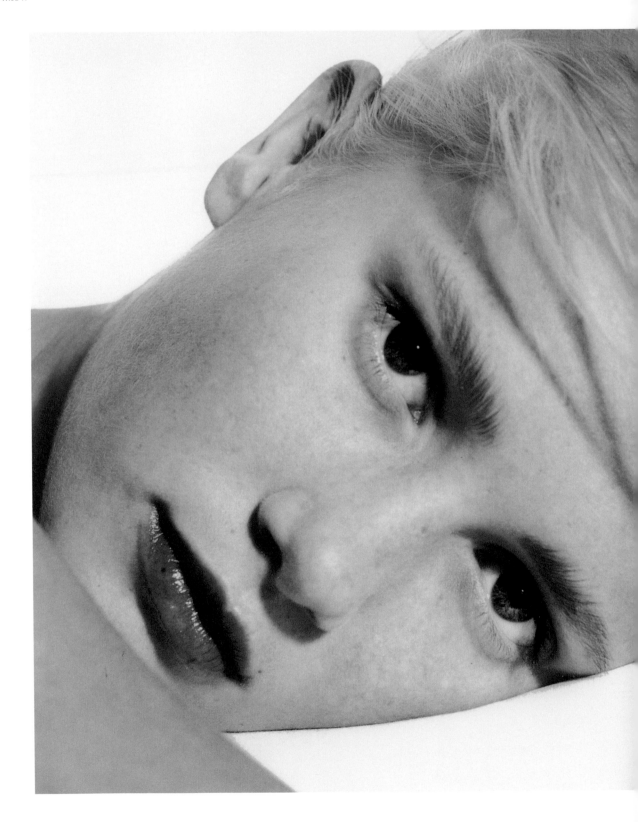

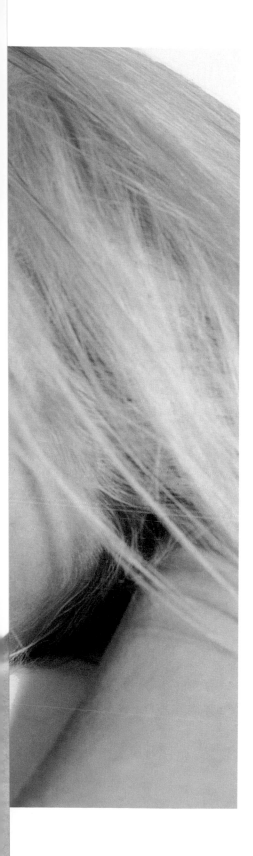

■ THERE ARE TWO WAYS OF APPLYING COLOUR, AND THAT'S WITH A PENCIL OR AN EYE SHADOW APPLIED WITH A BRUSH. WHICH YOU CHOOSE DEPENDS ON THE EFFECT YOU WANT TO ACHIEVE.

■ WHEN YOU PUT ON COLOUR, WHETHER WITH A PENCIL OR A BRUSH, APPLY IT IN SHORT SHARP STROKES SO THAT IT BLENDS IN WITH THE HAIR. THE MORE YOU APPLY, THE MORE DENSE THE COLOUR WILL BECOME. IN THIS WAY YOU CAN ACTUALLY GET A VARIETY OF COLOUR FROM THE SAME PRODUCT.

■ IF YOU HAVE PLUCKED YOUR EYEBROWS AND DON'T HAVE A LOT OF HAIR, USE A PENCIL BECAUSE POWDER NEEDS THE HAIR TO STICK TO. YOU CAN ALWAYS BLEND PENCIL WITH A BRUSH AFTERWARDS TO MAKE IT LOOK MORE NATURAL. AND ALWAYS BLEND UPWARDS IN THE DIRECTION OF THE HAIR GROWTH.

applying

eyebrow

colour

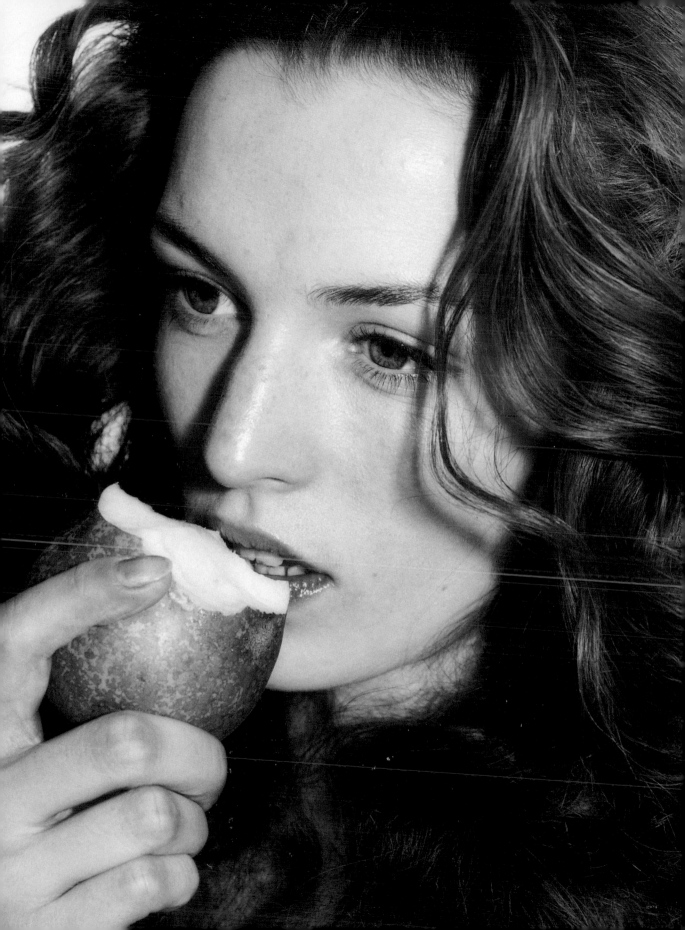

contour and highlight

'THE TWO GOLDEN RULES ARE: HIGHLIGHT REFLECTS LIGHT, BRINGING AN AREA FORWARD, WHILE CONTOUR IS DARK, SO CONCEALS AND PUSHES AN AREA BACK.'

Although contour and highlight are very important, it is not perceived as being very modern. However, you will find that contour and highlight crop up all over your face; whether you are doing it intentionally or not. It doesn't just apply to the face and cheekbones; in fact, we use eye shadow to contour and highlight, lip colour even. When you use dark and light colours on the eyes you are highlighting and contouring.

It is all about shade and light, but isn't nearly as complicated as it seems – unless you're going in for hard-core contouring that is, which really should be left to the professionals. Look at your natural highlight and contour, look at the areas that naturally come forward and catch the light and the ones that naturally recess and don't catch the light.

For example, the area around the base of your nose is dark but you can lighten it to get rid of dark shadows. If your cheekbones are not catching as much light as you would like them to (making them look more prominent), add a touch of highlight to bring them forward. You may find that the end of your nose comes out

too much and with a little bit of muted colour on the tip you can push it back. There might be days when you wake up and your eyes are more sunken, so then you can use a light concealer to even out the darkness, but you might need a touch of white shimmery powder to bring the area forward. Highlight does not have to be luminescent or shimmery, it just needs to be paler than the area you're highlighting. And remember that light attracts light, so when you go out, anything you have highlighted will stand out even more, so be prepared.

When it comes to contouring, although this is a rather old-fashioned technique, it's something that Millie swears by.

● Using a taupe coloured powder, brush under the cheekbone, down the lower cheek area (under your blusher) and under the jaw line in a triangle shape underneath the chin.

● This gives the illusion of lift under the chin and accentuates bone structure.

● Millie suggests you concentrate on your cheeks and eyebrows during the day, but this is a brilliant trick that works just as well in evening or false light.

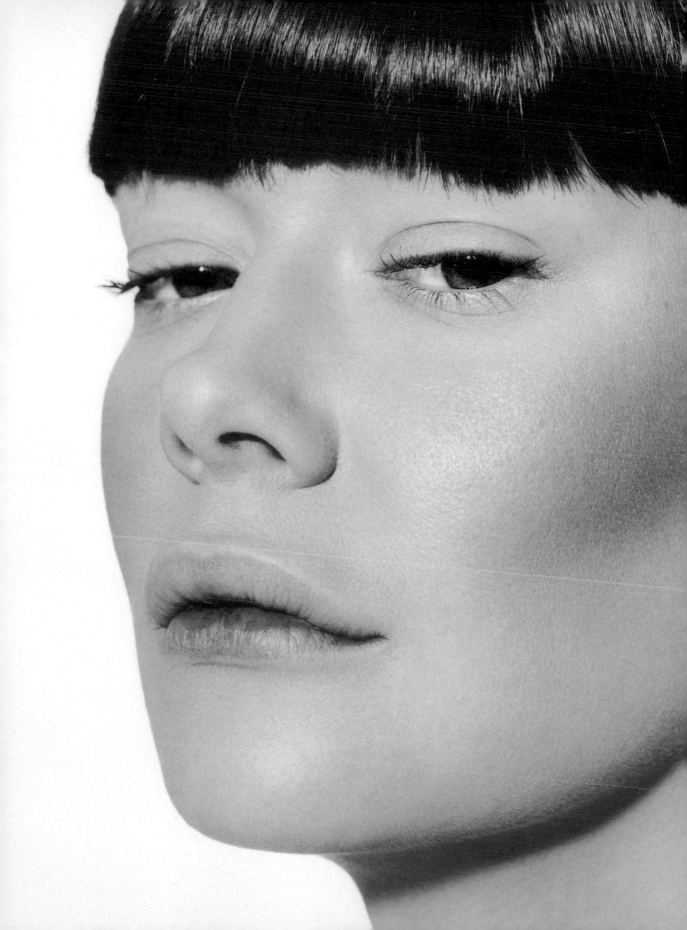

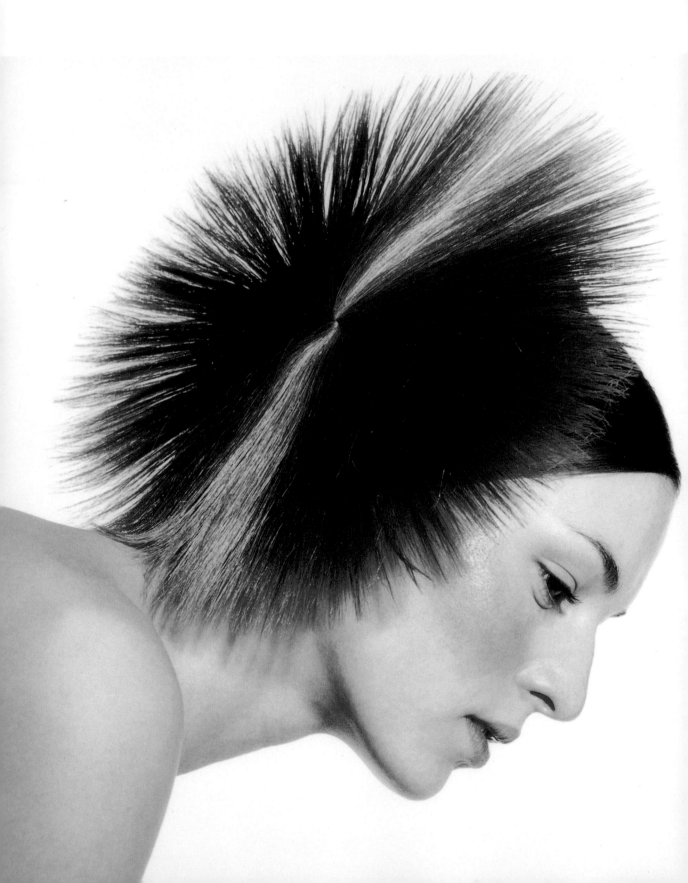

cheeky colour

A flush of colour really does boost the face. We swear by cheek colour, it makes you look refreshed, revived and sexy. But the cheeks are often forgotten. We tend to put a lot of emphasis on our lips and eyes, but the cheeks are just as important.

Get to know your cheekbones. Looking in the mirror, take your middle finger and put it on the top of the cheekbone and follow it down to where it finishes. Where do you naturally blush, because ideally this is where your colour should go? Nobody blushes up the side of their face where their eyes are or along the hairline.

Whether to go for powder, cream or gel is, of course, entirely your choice. Usually cream and gel are put on with the fingers and powder is best applied with a brush. But what colour is the best? In the past you might have wanted a monochromatic colour to tone in with the rest of your make-up, but those days are long gone and every rule on that front has been broken. Nowadays a slight flush of orange on the cheeks with a vibrant pink lipstick can look stunning. Any colour goes, whether iridescent or matte.

● There may be times when orange will make you look more lively and fresh.

● Or a rose tone will make you look a bit more sophisticated, whereas peach is more youthful. Again it comes down to the mood you want to express, as well as your skin colouring.

● It might be that on yellow-toned skin, anything pinky is a contrast and peach shades blend well and match better. Decide whether to complement or contrast.

● Using a pink tone on pale skin can look very natural but on a darker or olive skin it would look completely unnatural.

Work with both your skin tone and the cosmetic effect you want to achieve. Also look at your face and decide whether your cheek colour is going to be a predominant feature or blend in with the rest of your make-up, and then you will be guided by what colour to use and how much.

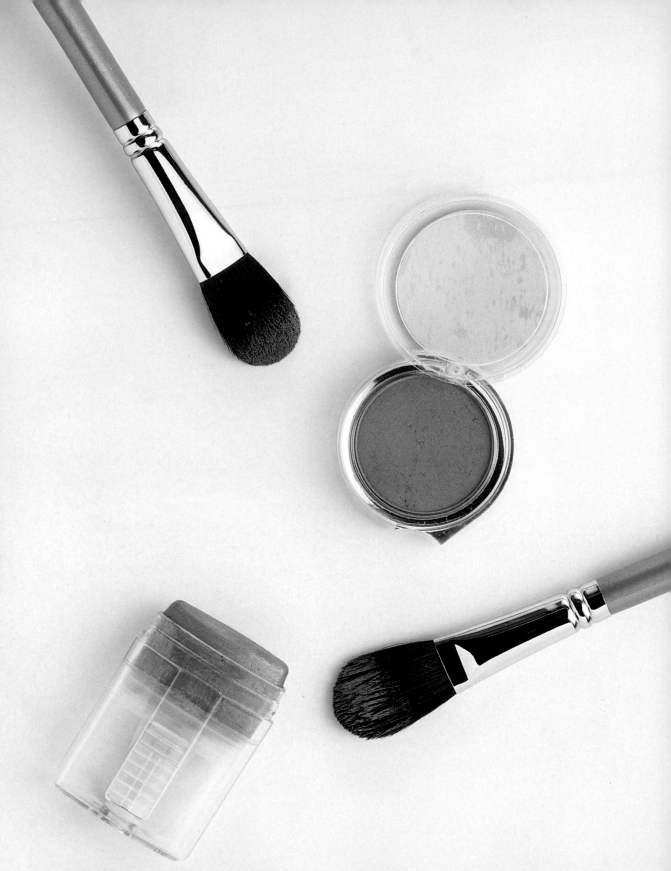

APPLYING CHEEK COLOUR

■ THE FIRST THING TO REMEMBER IS THAT WHEN USING A CREAM OR GEL BLUSHER, PUT IT ON TOP OF YOUR BASE BEFORE YOU APPLY YOUR LOOSE POWDER.

■ IF YOU'RE USING POWDER BLUSHER, IT GOES ON TOP OF YOUR POWDER. BETTER STILL, DO BOTH AND YOUR CHEEK COLOUR WILL LAST MUCH LONGER.

■ THE MOST COMMON MISTAKE WHEN IT COMES TO BLUSHER, IS BEING TOO HEAVY-HANDED. TOO STRONG A COLOUR WITH TOO LARGE A BRUSH AND YES, YOU'LL BE LOOKING MORE LIKE A CLOWN THAN A FLUSHED BEAUTY.

■ A MAKE-UP ARTIST WILL USE A SMALLER BRUSH, SHIMMY IT BACK AND FORTH IN THE COLOUR TO GET A GOOD AMOUNT ON THE BRUSH, AND DUST OFF THE EXCESS ON TO A TISSUE BEFORE APPLYING IT TO THE FACE.

■ ONCE SHE HAS APPLIED HER COLOUR RUBY ALWAYS GOES OVER THE EDGE – WHETHER THE COLOUR IS NONDESCRIPT OR STRONGER – USING A CLEAN BRUSH OR A POWDER PUFF DIPPED IN TRANSLUCENT POWDER. IT JUST REFINES THE EDGES BECAUSE NOBODY BLUSHES IN SHAPES OR STRIPES.

■ GETTING THE RIGHT BRUSH IS IMPORTANT. THE BIGGER THE BRUSH THE MORE COLOUR YOU'RE PUTTING ON TO YOUR FACE. MILLIE'S TIP FOR TESTING A BRUSH FOR SIZE IS TO HOLD IT OVER YOUR CHEEK AND PRESS IT ON TO YOUR FACE. SEE HOW MUCH IT SPLAYS OUT AND THAT IS WHERE YOU WILL GET YOUR COLOUR.

■ A BRUSH THAT'S TOO BIG WILL COVER THE WHOLE CHEEK AREA, AND ONE THAT'S TOO SMALL WILL GIVE YOU THIN STRIPES OF COLOUR.

■ CHOOSE A MEDIUM-SIZED BRUSH, BIG ENOUGH TO COVER THE APPLE OF THE CHEEK, AND YOU'LL END UP WITH A MUCH MORE CONTROLLED AREA OF BLUSHER.

■ WHEN APPLYING THE COLOUR WITH A BRUSH, DO NOT DAB THE BRISTLES HEAD-ON TOWARDS YOUR FACE. AS WELL AS CREATING A HOLE IN THE MIDDLE OF YOUR BRUSH, YOU'LL ALSO END UP WITH A CIRCLE OF BLUSHER ON YOUR CHEEK.

■ PUT THE BRUSH FLAT ON YOUR CHEEK (APPLE OR CHEEKBONE) AND WORK IT BACKWARDS TOWARDS THE OUTER EDGE OF YOUR FACE. APART FROM NOT DAMAGING YOUR BRUSH, YOU GET A NICER BLENDED LOOK.

■ AS THE BRUSH HITS THE FACE MOST OF THE COLOUR IS DISPENSED HERE, SO THIS IS WHERE YOU WILL GET THE MOST INTENSITY OF COLOUR. WHEN USING YOUR FINGERS, USE THE SAME PRINCIPLE BUT BLEND THE COLOUR IN VERY GENTLY WITH YOUR FINGERTIPS.

eyes up

'THE EYES AND LIPS ARE THE TWO MOST MOBILE AREAS OF THE FACE, AND THEREFORE THE MOST EXPRESSIVE. AND BECAUSE THEY ARE SO EXPRESSIVE THEY CAN CONVEY A LOT OF DIFFERENT MESSAGES, WHETHER THEY'RE STRONG AND DRAMATIC OR SUBTLE AND DEMURE. WE ALL HAVE DIFFERENT EYE COLOURS AND DIFFERENT HAIR COLOUR BUT THERE ARE REALLY NO HARD-AND-FAST RULES WHEN IT COMES TO PUTTING COLOUR ON THE EYES. THE EYE IS MADE UP OF COLOUR, SHAPE, WIDTH AND DEPTH, AND WITHIN THAT, USING THE RIGHT TOOLS, YOU CAN CONVEY WHATEVER MESSAGE YOU LIKE.'

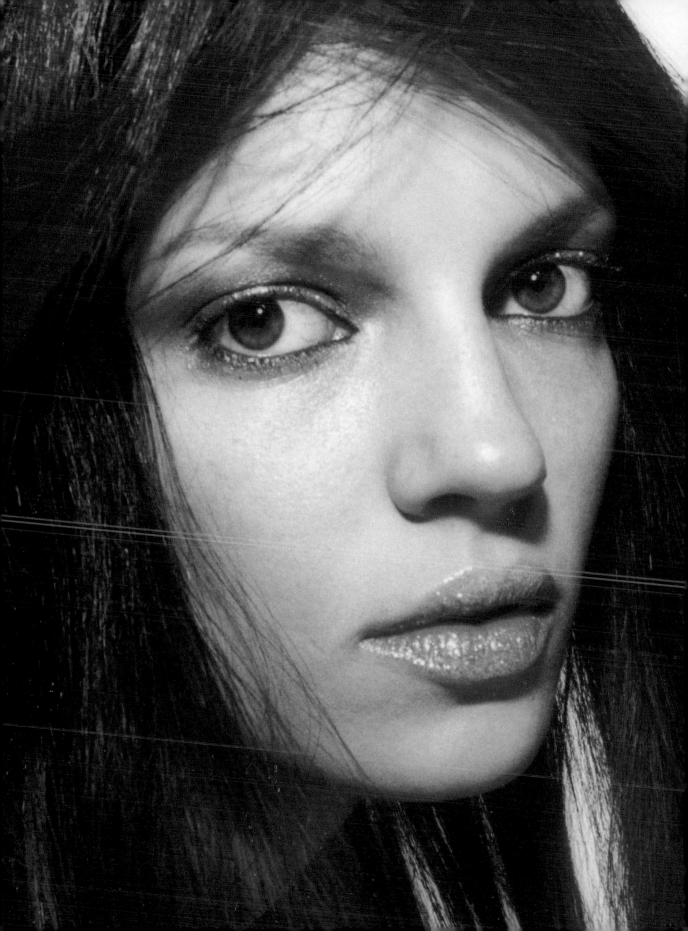

eye

shadow

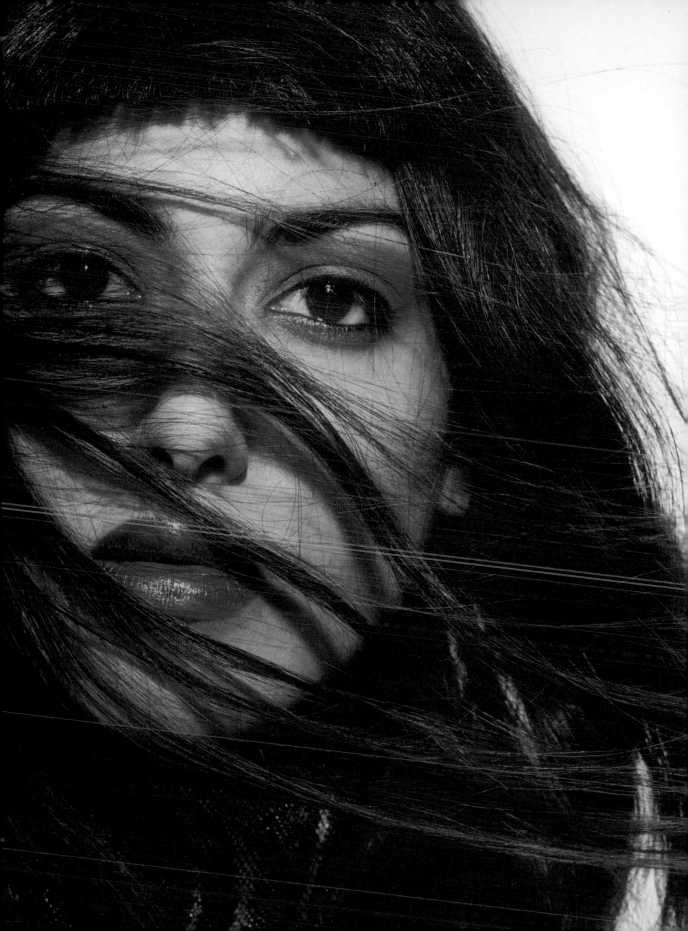

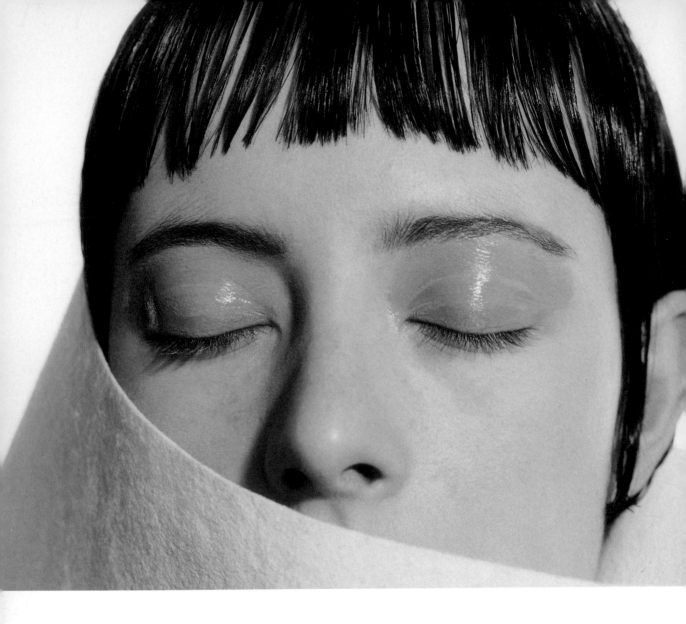

accentuate the positive

When choosing eye colour, do you want to complement your eyes or create something with a bit more drama? There will be times when you want to draw attention to your eyes and times when you don't. There are three types of colour:

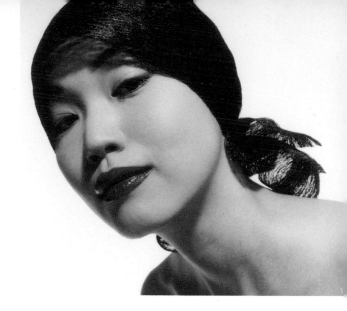

- pale, highlight colours,
- mid-tones for basic lid work,
- and stronger shades.

There was a time when women felt they had to use all three on their eyes, then eye colour went monochrome. But now anything goes. It can be one colour for maximum impact or five colours blended together to look like nothing. The choice is yours.

One way of introducing yourself to colour is by using a neutral base colour (mid-tone) – beige, taupe, mushroom, mink, khaki – and then apply a stronger colour in the crease over the top. Many women are frightened of moving away from the beiges and taupes; they are comfortable and easy to wear after all. To explore and experiment with colour, Millie suggests applying your mid-tone on the eyelid or in the crease of the eye, and add just a touch of colour, whether it be a thin stripe, a little in the corner or a wash of colour over the top. Build up the colour gradually and see if you like it.

Some colours look vibrant in the palette but much more subtle once applied to the skin. It also depends on your application and how heavy-handed you are. Are you taking a very strong colour and blending it, or are you leaving it as it is for maximum impact? It's down to you. The great thing about eye shadow is that you can put it on and take it off, you don't ever have to be stuck with something you don't like.

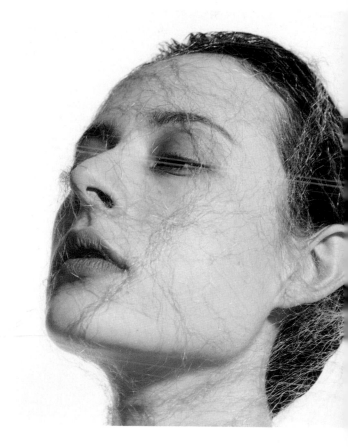

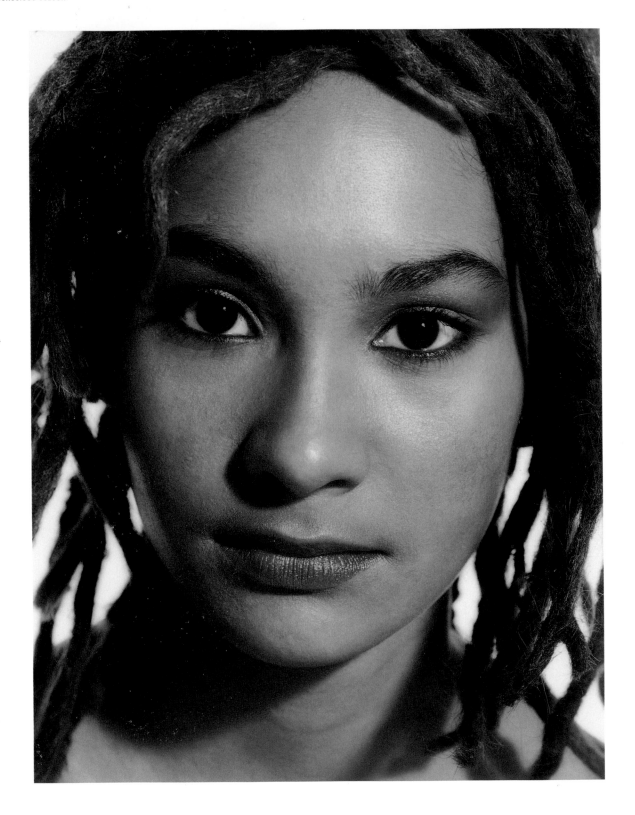

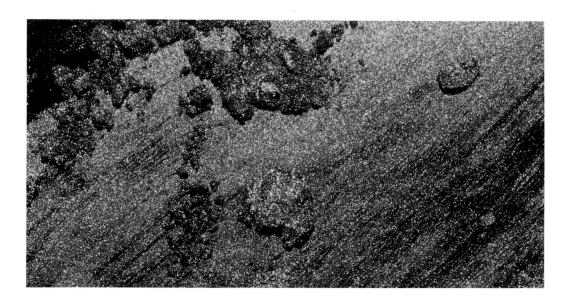

eye shadow formulations

Be aware of the formulations of eye shadow that are available for you to experiment with.

● Highlight can either be matte or slightly iridescent. You would normally put it on the brow bone or all over the eyelid. It's usually quite sheer so that it can be blended in very easily, giving you a bare-skinned effect with a hint of shimmer.

● The same shades in a matte formula will look more like nude skin.

● Mid-tones are usually slightly heavier in consistency and again they can be matte or shimmer. They're still muted and easy to blend but they are there to be seen.

● If you're unsure about bright colour, try deeper tones instead, such as blues and greens. A forest green may not be a bright plant green but it will certainly be darker and stronger. This is also where you can add real sparkle, so instead of shimmer you get more of a frost. And then you have the choice of powder or cream eye shadow.

● With creams you can either wear them alone, with powder eye shadow, or with loose powder on top. Cream on its own will look glossy and very sexy.

● With loose powder on top you will have a more subtle colour (less dense than powder eye shadow) but with great staying power. Powder eye shadow over the top will give you a really strong vibrant colour, but once the powder is on it's very hard to blend.

To see which you prefer, Millie suggests putting a cream colour on the back of your hand, adding loose powder to half of it and powder eye shadow to the other half.

EYE SHADOW TOOLS

■ TOOLS FOR POWDER. WHEN CHOOSING YOUR BRUSHES LOOK OUT FOR ONES WITH SABLE HAIR, WHICH ARE THE BEST QUALITY AND DISTRIBUTE POWDER BRILLIANTLY.

■ SYNTHETIC BRUSHES WORK MUCH BETTER WITH CREAM FORMULATIONS.

■ RUBY STRONGLY BELIEVES IN HAVING MORE THAN ONE BRUSH FOR YOUR EYE SHADOW. IF YOU'RE GOING TO USE MORE THAN ONE COLOUR AND YOU'RE DIPPING THE BRUSH IN AND OUT OF DIFFERENT SHADES, YOU WILL NOT GET THE TRUE COLOUR ON YOUR BRUSH.

■ IDEALLY, YOU NEED A MINIMUM OF TWO BRUSHES: ONE TO DEPOSIT YOUR MID-TONES AND THE OTHER FOR DARKER SHADES.

■ IF YOU CAN AFFORD IT, THREE IS EVEN BETTER SO YOU CAN HAVE A CLEAN ONE FOR HIGHLIGHTING.

■ THERE ARE ALSO DIFFERENT SHAPES AVAILABLE – ONE COULD BE THINNER AND THE OTHER MORE DIFFUSED FOR BLENDING.

■ THE BEST EYE SHADOW BRUSHES ARE SHAPED WITH A GENEROUS DOME – THE OUTSIDE BRISTLES SHOULD BE SHORTER THAN THE ONES IN THE CENTRE. THIS WILL ENABLE THE BRUSH TO BLEND FOR YOU.

■ LARGER BRUSHES ARE BETTER FOR LIGHTER SHADES BECAUSE THEY SWEEP OVER A WIDER AREA. USE MEDIUM-SIZED BRUSHES FOR THE MID-TONES AND SMALLER FOR DARKER TONES AND DEFINITION.

■ IF THE ONE BRUSH REALLY IS YOUR LIMIT, RUBY HAS A BRILLIANT TIP. WHEN APPLYING YOUR EYE SHADOW KEEP YOUR TRANSLUCENT POWDER ON HAND. WHEN YOU ARE BLENDING, USING THE SAME BRUSH WILL JUST KEEP DEPOSITING MORE COLOUR ON TO YOUR SKIN. BUT IF YOU DIP THE BRUSH INTO YOUR LOOSE POWDER IT ALLOWS YOU TO BLEND WITHOUT ADDING ANY MORE COLOUR OR STRENGTH. THE POWDER IS ALSO GREAT FOR CLEANING AND SMOOTHING AROUND THE EDGES.

■ TOOLS FOR CREAM. SABLE IS FANTASTIC FOR POWDER EYE SHADOW BUT BECAUSE THE HAIRS ARE SO DENSE AND THICK, IT WILL LEAVE A STREAKY EFFECT IF YOU USE A SABLE BRUSH WITH CREAM SHADOW.

■ A SYNTHETIC BRUSH WILL BLEND CREAM MUCH MORE EASILY. ALTERNATIVELY, YOU CAN USE YOUR FINGERS, APPLYING THE CREAM LITTLE BY LITTLE.

■ WHEN WE HAVE A CHOICE, WE PREFER USING A BRUSH INSTEAD OF FINGERS BECAUSE IT'S CLEANER AND MORE HYGIENIC, AND, APART FROM ANYTHING ELSE, BRUSHES ARE DESIGNED TO BLEND, MAKING THE JOB EASIER.

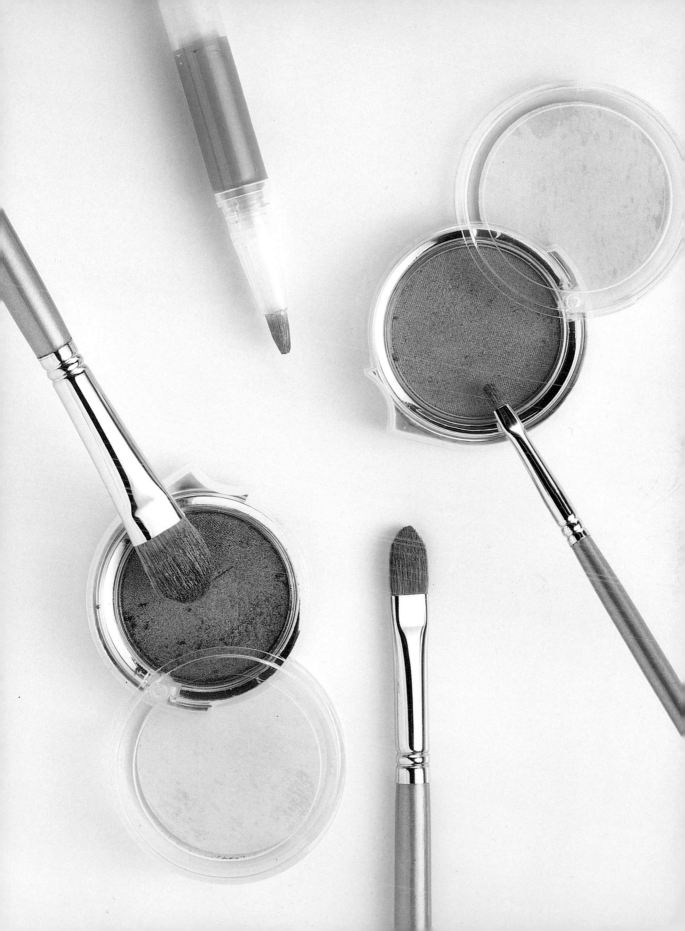

APPLYING EYE COLOUR

■ WHATEVER YOU'RE APPLYING TO YOUR EYES, NEVER JUST PUT IT ON AND LEAVE IT THERE. SPEND PLENTY OF TIME APPLYING THE COLOUR AND BLENDING IT UP OR DOWN.

■ BLENDING IS THE DONKEY-WORK OF MAKE-UP. THE RIGHT COLOUR SLOPPED ON WITH THE RIGHT TOOL IS NOT ENOUGH, HOWEVER AMAZING THE FORMULA. THERE IS NO PRECISE SCIENCE TO THE APPLICATION OF EYE SHADOW. JUST MAKE SURE YOU HAVE THE RIGHT TOOLS AND LET THEM DO THE WORK FOR YOU.

■ WHEN A MAKE-UP ARTIST APPLIES EYE SHADOW THEY USUALLY DO THE BASE COLOUR FIRST, WHETHER IT BE LIGHT OR MID-TONE, AND THEN APPLY THE DEFINITION.

■ HOWEVER, MILLIE, WHO FINDS SHE'S VERY SLOPPY WHEN IT COMES TO STRONGER COLOURS, DOES IT THE OPPOSITE WAY ROUND. SHE PUTS HER DARKER COLOUR ON FIRST, AND THEN USES HER MID-TONE OR HIGHLIGHTER TO BLEND IT OUT.

■ SO HOW DO YOU APPLY THAT FIRST DROP OF COLOUR? EVEN RUBY FINDS IT UNNERVING AT TIMES, HER TIP IS TO TAKE YOUR BRUSH WITH THE COLOUR (DUST OFF THE EXCESS), AND INSTEAD OF CLOSING YOUR EYES, LOOK STRAIGHT AHEAD,

■ HOLD THE BRUSH FLAT ON THE OUTER CORNER OF YOUR EYE AND WITH ONE SMOOTH MOVEMENT JUST LET IT MOVE FREELY ALONG THE CREASE OF THE EYE. YOU CAN THEN FILL IN THE GAPS, TRUST THAT THE BRUSH IS GOING TO DO THE WORK AND IT SHOULD COME OUT PERFECTLY.

■ WHEN IT COMES TO EYES, OUR PHILOSOPHY IS BLEND, BLEND, BLEND. AND WHEN YOU THINK YOU HAVE DONE ENOUGH, BLEND SOME MORE. WHAT YOU WILL END UP WITH IS A SMOOTH PROFESSIONAL FINISH.

■ YOU DON'T WANT ANY SHARP LINES WHERE ONE COLOUR STARTS AND ANOTHER FINISHES, YOU WANT A SMOOTH AND BALANCED WASH. WHEN MILLIE HAS WATCHED MAKE-UP ARTISTS APPLYING EYE SHADOW, MOST OF THE BLENDING IS DONE ON THE OUTER HALF OF THE EYE, BLENDING INWARDS TO SOFTEN THE EDGES.

■ BE WARNED: ANYTHING TOO DARK ON THE INSIDE OF YOUR EYE NEAR THE NOSE BRINGS YOUR EYES CLOSER TOGETHER.

■ EVEN IF YOU'RE WEARING BRIGHT GARISH COLOURS YOU WANT THEM TO WORK WITH THE NATURAL CONTOUR OF THE EYE. IF YOU LOOK AT YOUR EYES WITHOUT MAKE-UP ON, THAT IS THE SHAPE YOU WANT BUT WITH ADDED COLOUR.

■ WE DON'T BELIEVE IN YOUR EYE SHAPE DETERMINING YOUR EYE MAKE-UP, BUT BECAUSE WE ARE ALL DIFFERENT, BE REALISTIC ABOUT YOUR EXPECTATIONS.

■ REMEMBER, THE EYE AREA INCLUDES ABOVE AND BELOW YOUR EYEBALL. A LOT OF PEOPLE FORGET TO JOIN THEM UP, THEY MAY DO IT WITH EYELINER BUT RARELY EYE SHADOW.

■ IF YOU ARE WEARING A BRIGHT COLOUR ON YOUR EYELIDS, TAKE A MID-TONE AROUND UNDER THE EYE. ALWAYS FINISH OFF UNDER THE EYE OR IT WILL LOOK TOP HEAVY.

■ KEEP A POT OF Q-TIPS ON HAND. DIPPED INTO TRANSLUCENT POWDER THEY ARE A GREAT TOOL FOR SOFTENING ANY HARD EDGES AND WIPING AWAY MISTAKES.

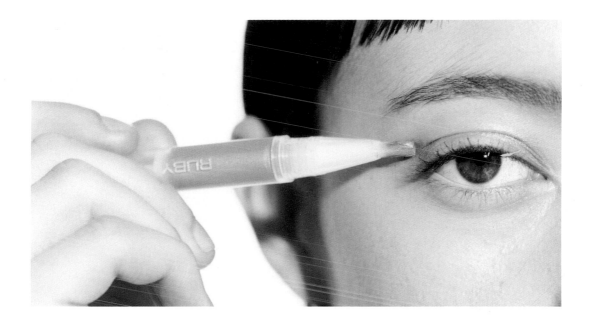

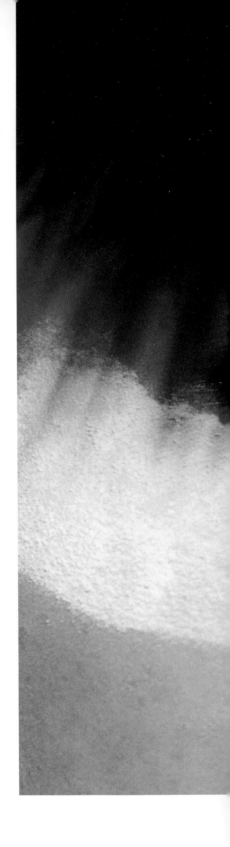

WHEN APPLYING EYE SHADOW, DAB ON A FAIRLY THICK COATING OF TRANSLUCENT POWDER UNDER THE CRESCENT AREA OF YOUR EYE TO COLLECT ANY DEPOSITS OF EYE SHADOW THAT FALL DOWN. WHISK AWAY WITH A BRUSH WHEN YOU HAVE FINISHED BLENDING. THIS AVOIDS ANY BLOBS OR SMEARS. THIS PHOTOGRAPH IS A GREATLY EXAGGERATED EXAMPLE OF THIS TECHNIQUE – WHAT AN EFFECT.

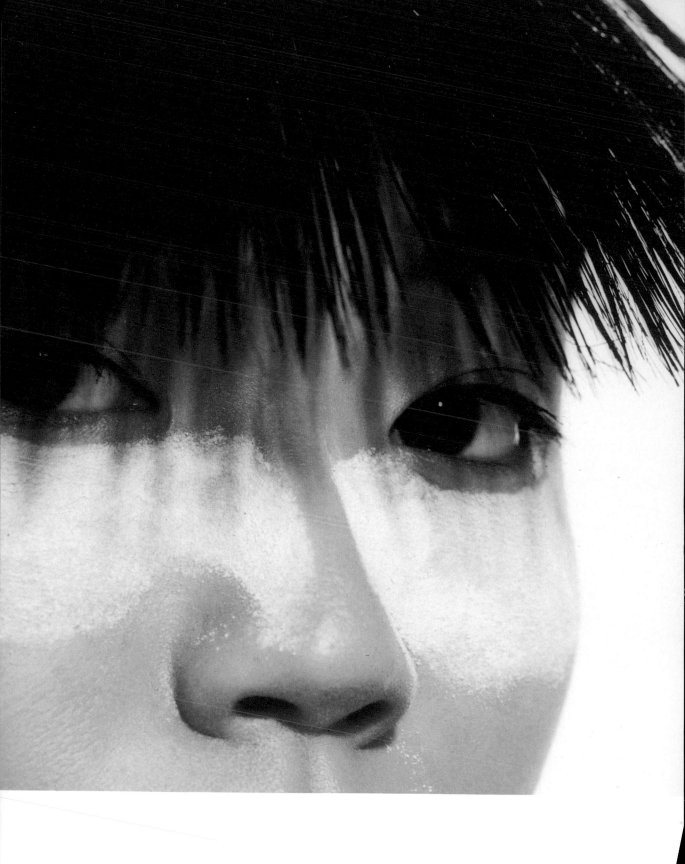

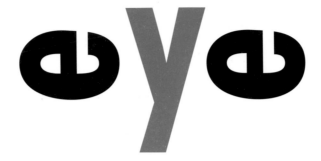

Eyeliner was originally invented for defining the lashes and making them look fuller. Now it is used to create more impact. It can certainly turn a day into a night and redefine your make-up in a few seconds. The formulation of eyeliner makes that job easier for you whether it be a pencil, felt pen, liquid or cake liner. You could sit there for hours with an eye shadow, and yes you would get a line along the top lashes as well as plenty of speckles and gunky bits underneath the eye. Eyeliner just makes the job clean and simple.

Lining the eyes is about depositing a very fine layer of colour right at the base of the eyelashes. It can help make the eyes appear whiter and push the iris out, you don't necessarily want it to have an eyeliner effect. Instead of using black, which most of us are so familiar with, use a natural-looking mid-to-deep tone colour for this or something to match your eye shadow. It makes the lashes look more defined and the eyes cleaner.

We are great fans of applying eyeliner on the inside of the eye. The rule has always been that anything you put on the inside of your eye will close it up, but this does not have to be the case. It works for Millie because she has big eyes and it makes them look longer and thinner. Ruby has smaller eyes and yes, technically, it probably does close them up, but she likes the aura of mystery it gives her.

You don't always have to use a dark colour either; Millie loves light green or a touch of shimmer. If you want an innocent, wide-eyed look then stay away from this area, but if you're looking for something edgy and sexy it works. But do keep in mind that it will not last. Either keep reapplying or let it smudge under the eye, which can also look very sexy. Again, it's a taste thing.

liner

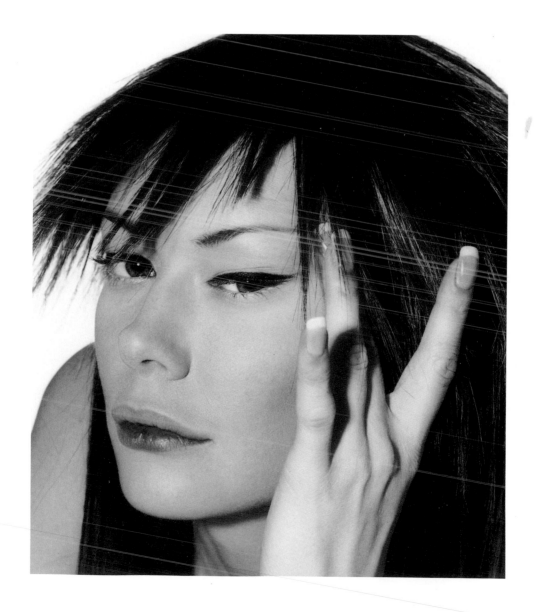

APPLYING EYELINER

■ THE IDIOT-PROOF WAY TO APPLY EYELINER IS TO START FROM THE OUTSIDE CORNER AND WORK YOUR WAY IN.

■ IF YOU CLOSE ONE EYE AND LOOK AT YOUR EYELID, YOU WILL SEE THAT YOU HAVE TINY LITTLE LINES THAT GO DOWN INTO THE EYELASH – AND WHAT YOU DON'T WANT TO DO IS GO AGAINST THEM. FOLLOW THE LINES AND WORK WITH THE GRAIN OF THE EYELID.

■ MILLIE APPLIES HER EYELINER IN LITTLE SECTIONS BECAUSE SHE CAN'T DRAW ONE LONG LINE. SHE FINDS IT EASIER TO APPLY SHORT STROKES AND BLEND THEM TOGETHER AFTERWARDS WITH A SMALL BRUSH.

■ DON'T START DIRECTLY ON THE LASH LINE BUT SLOPE SLIGHTLY UPWARDS. IF YOU FOLLOW THE LASH LINE FROM THE VERY BEGINNING, WHEN YOU OPEN YOUR EYE YOUR EYELINER WILL SLANT DOWNWARDS, GIVING YOU DOWN-TURNED EYES.

■ START WITH A SLIGHT KICK, NOT THE CLEOPATRA KIND, JUST ENOUGH TO LIFT UP THE CORNER OF THE EYE. THE GREAT THING ABOUT EYELINER IS THAT YOU CAN BLEND AND SOFTEN IT BEFORE IT DRIES. YOU DON'T HAVE TO HAVE A STRONG, DRAMATIC LINE.

■ TAKE TIME TO PRACTISE WITH EYELINER. IF YOU ARE DOING IT FOR THE FIRST TIME YOU DON'T WANT TO BE SHORT OF TIME OR ON YOUR WAY OUT. IT'S SUCH AN INTRICATE THING FOR A MAKE-UP ARTIST, LET ALONE DOING IT YOURSELF.

■ ALWAYS KEEP YOUR ELBOW STEADY BY BALANCING IT ON A SURFACE IF YOU CAN, OTHERWISE TUCK IT INTO YOUR WAIST FOR SUPPORT.

■ BE PREPARED TO CLEAN UP A LITTLE AFTERWARDS BECAUSE EVEN IF YOU HAVE THE STEADIEST HANDS IN THE WORLD IT'S VERY EASY TO GO OFF COURSE SLIGHTLY. RUBY USES A TINY AMOUNT OF CONCEALER TO CLEAN THE LINES UP SO THEY ARE NICE AND SMOOTH.

■ TO MAKE THE COLOUR OR LINE EVEN DENSER, TRACE ALONG THE LINE WITH A POWDER EYE SHADOW. IT WILL ALSO MAKE IT LONGER LASTING.

■ ALWAYS SHARPEN YOUR PENCIL BEFORE YOU USE IT (MILLIE DOES IT AFTER SHE'S USED IT) SO IT IS READY FOR THE NEXT TIME,

■ LOOK OUT FOR SOFT PENCILS THAT DON'T DRAG OVER THE EYE AND SCRATCH. STAY AWAY FROM VERY HARD ONES.

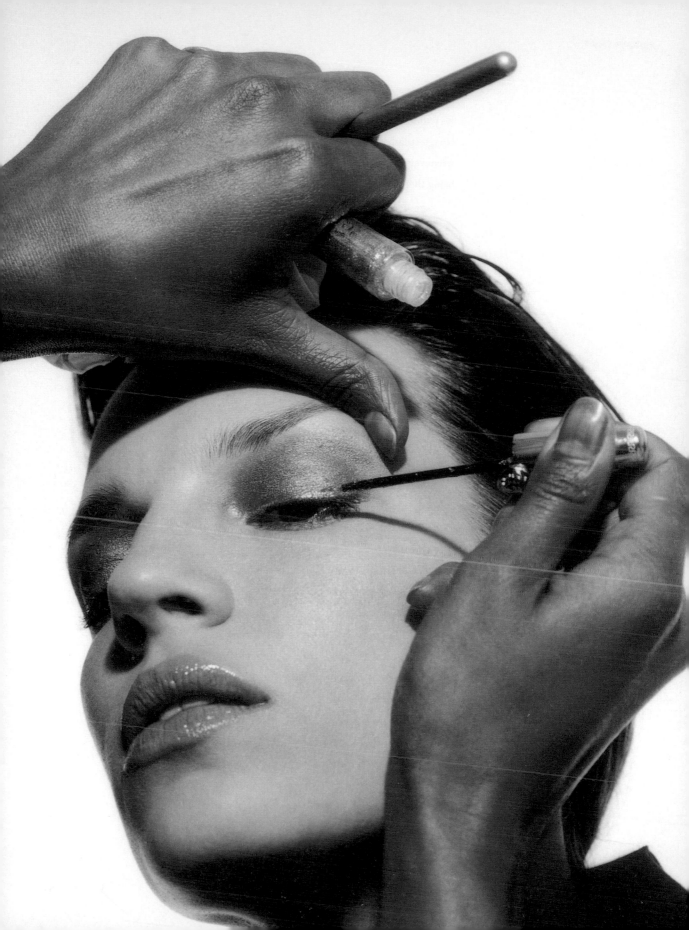

APPLYING MASCARA

■ APPLY PLENTY OF THIN LAYERS, LETTING THEM DRY IN BETWEEN. MILLIE PUTS MOST OF HER MASCARA ON THE OUTER EDGES OF HER
EYE SO THAT THE LASHES FAN OUT MORE. LOOK UP WHEN DOING YOUR LOWER LASHES, AND LOOK DOWN WHEN DOING THE UPPER ONES.

■ IF RUBY HAS APPLIED A LOT OF EYE SHADOW BEFOREHAND, SHE LIKES TO APPLY THE MASCARA FROM THE ROOT TO THE TIP ON TOP OF
THE LASHES TO COVER UP ANY LOOSE POWDER THAT MIGHT BE THERE, AND THEN SHE APPLIES MORE UNDERNEATH.

■ IF YOU WANT TO WEAR MASCARA ON THE BOTTOM LASHES – AND NOT EVERYONE DOES – DO THEM FIRST. IF YOU DON'T DO THIS, THE
NEWLY APPLIED MASCARA ON THE TOP LASHES IS GOING TO LEAVE DOTS ON YOUR UPPER EYELID.

■ DON'T SHARE YOUR MASCARA WITH ANYBODY AND THROW IT AWAY AFTER ABOUT THREE MONTHS. PUMPING THE WAND LETS IN
BACTERIA AND ALSO DRIES OUT THE PRODUCT.

■ IF YOU DO MAKE A MISTAKE WITH YOUR MASCARA, WHATEVER YOU DON'T RUB IT WITH YOUR FINGER. DIP A Q-TIP INTO YOUR
FOUNDATION AND GENTLY WIPE AWAY THE SMUDGE.

■ USE A HEATED TEASPOON TO CURL YOUR LASHES BEFORE APPLYING MASCARA.

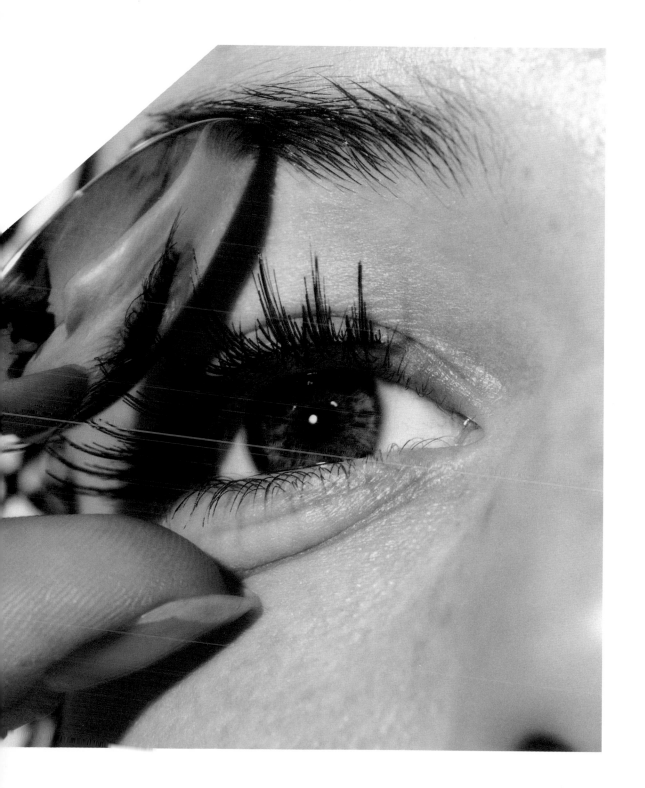

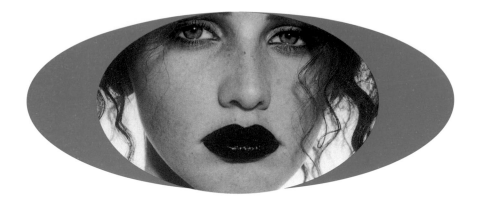

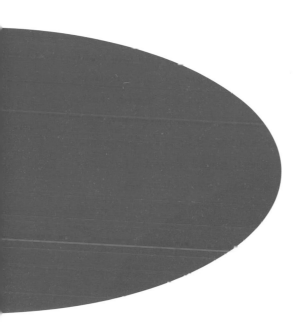

lip tips

'IT DOESN'T MATTER WHAT SHAPE YOUR LIPS ARE, OR WHAT PRODUCT YOU USE, WHAT YOU WANT IS AN INVITING, COLOURFUL MOUTH. LIPS EXPRESS MOTION AND MOOD, THEY'RE ALWAYS ON THE GO. WHETHER IT'S A BRIGHT GLOSSY RED OR A SOMBRE BROWN, LIP COLOUR EXPRESSES OUR CHARACTER OF THE MOMENT. GLOSS, MATTE, SHEER OR PENCIL, WE USE AN ARRAY OF PRODUCTS AND HUGE AMOUNTS OF COLOUR DURING OUR LIFETIME. USE IT TO YOUR ADVANTAGE.'

There is no shortage of colour, so what we suggest is that you try something from each colour family. It's very simple, they include red, pink, orange, purple, brown and beige. Choose one that's right for you from each group. For example, from the orange family you could have one that's almost brown but with an orange base, which might look better on one skin tone than another. A lot of make-up artists blend these families together too and with a bit of experimenting there's no reason why you shouldn't either.

● Pinks and purples blend well together, as do the reds, pinks and oranges.

● You can take a red and make it more orange or pink.

● You can make a brown more orange or beige.

● Then you have your cool (bluer) and warm (more orange) tones. If a purple has more pink in it, it's cooler, but a purple going towards brown will be slightly warmer.

● An orange red is warm whereas a purple red is cool.

● Warmer tones are more user-friendly, but you'll only find what tones work best for you by playing and experimenting.

Because of the nature of lipstick – it's waxy and creamy – you can blend colours together very easily. You almost can't go wrong. If you don't feel confident blending directly on your lips, do it on the base of your hand first.

colour families

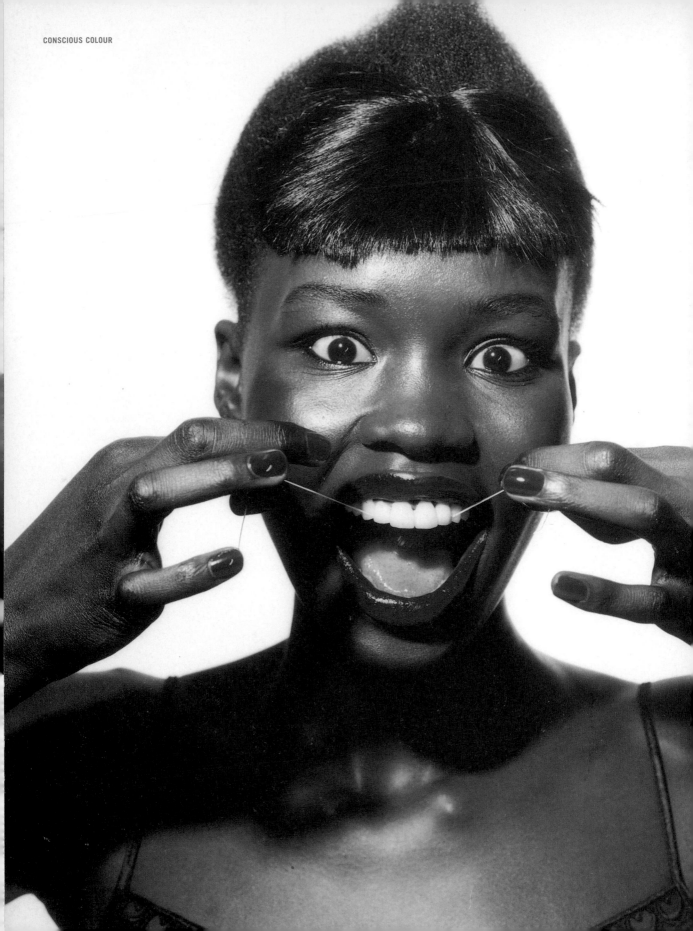

CREATING LONG-LASTING LIPS

■ IF YOU PICK A GLOSS, IT'S NOT GOING TO LAST AS LONG AS A MATTE LIPSTICK. ASSESS WHAT YOU WANT TO ACHIEVE FROM YOUR LIP COLOUR AND DON'T HAVE UNREALISTIC EXPECTATIONS. ARE YOU GOING TO THE CINEMA OR ARE YOU GOING OUT DRINKING AND EATING?

■ LIP GLOSS NEEDS REGULAR REAPPLYING, WHEREAS SOMETHING MATTE WILL PROBABLY ONLY NEED ONE TOUCH-UP. THE TEXTURE YOU CHOOSE WILL HAVE SOME BEARING ON HOW LONG YOUR COLOUR WILL LAST.

■ FOR LONG-LASTING COLOUR, LIKE YOUR SKIN, YOU WANT A NICE, SMOOTH BASE. DAB A LITTLE FOUNDATION, CONCEALER OR MIXTURE OF THE TWO ON TO YOUR LIPS.

■ A NUDE COLOURED LIP PENCIL WORKS JUST AS WELL. THIS SEALS THE EDGES AND STOPS THEM FROM BLEEDING, AS WELL AS GIVING THE COLOUR SOMETHING TO ADHERE TO.

■ APPLY A GOOD EVEN COATING OF COLOUR; YOU DON'T WANT IT TO COME OFF IN PATCHES, LIPSTICK SHOULD WEAR OFF EVENLY. APPLY ONE GOOD LAYER, AND THEN, USING A LAYER OF TISSUE, HOLD GENTLY OVER YOUR MOUTH AND BLOT.

■ YOU CAN ALSO DIP YOUR BRUSH INTO LOOSE POWDER AND DAB ON TO THE LIPS THROUGH THE TISSUE. THE TISSUE ACTS LIKE A SIEVE. ADD MORE COLOUR AND BLOT AGAIN, FINISHING WITH A FINAL LAYER OF COLOUR. BLOT AGAIN IF YOU WANT A MATTE LOOK. THE TRICK IS TO BUILD LOTS OF THIN, EVEN LAYERS OF COLOUR, INSTEAD OF ONE THICK, GLOOPY ONE.

■ LIPSTICKS THAT ARE MANUFACTURED AS 'LONG-LASTING' OFTEN TEND TO STICK TO THE EDGES OF THE LIPS AND FADE IN THE MIDDLE.

■ THE IDIOT'S GUIDE TO USING A LIP BRUSH: WHEN USING DARKER COLOURS, USE THE FLAT SIDE OF YOUR BRUSH AND DRAW A STRAIGHT LINE ALONG THE CENTRE OF YOUR BOTTOM LIP LINE. THIS IS THE FIRST DROP OF COLOUR, AND YOU CAN DECIDE IF YOU LIKE IT, OR WANT TO ADD TO IT OR MAKE IT MORE SUBTLE.

■ ADD TWO MORE LINES TO MAKE UP THE WHOLE BOTTOM LIP LINE, FROM THE CORNERS IN.

■ USING THE SAME TECHNIQUE FOR THE TOP LIP, LINE THE CUPID'S BOW, ONE SIDE AT A TIME, AND JOIN FROM THE CORNERS INWARDS AND UPWARDS. THEN WORK IN TOWARDS THE MIDDLE OF THE LIP. LIGHTER COLOURS SHOULD BE APPLIED FROM THE CENTRE OUT.

■ A DEFINITE LIP LINE WILL ONLY LOOK CHALKY. WHEN USING COLOUR STRAIGHT FROM THE TUBE, APPLY IN THE SAME WAY. LIP BRUSHES WERE DESIGNED TO SIMULATE YOUR FINGERS, THEY GIVE YOU MUCH MORE CONTROL, BUT DON'T GIVE YOURSELF TWO MINUTES BEFORE A PARTY, HAVE A PLAY WITH THEM ON YOUR NEXT EVENING IN.

■ REMEMBER THAT YOUR LIPS ARE CONSTANTLY ON THE MOVE AND UNLESS YOU INTEND TO SIT PERFECTLY STILL WITHOUT DRINKING, EATING OR TALKING, YOU WILL HAVE TO KEEP AN EYE ON YOUR LIPSTICK.

■ IF YOU SEE THE COLOUR SITTING ON THE EDGE OF YOUR LIPS – IT WILL LOOK AWFUL – TAKE THE WHOLE LOT OFF AND START AGAIN. YOU WILL HAVE TO GO TO THE TOILET AT SOME POINT IN THE EVENING, SO YOU MIGHT AS WELL DO YOUR LIPSTICK AT THE SAME TIME. IT WILL ONLY TAKE YOU A COUPLE OF MINUTES.

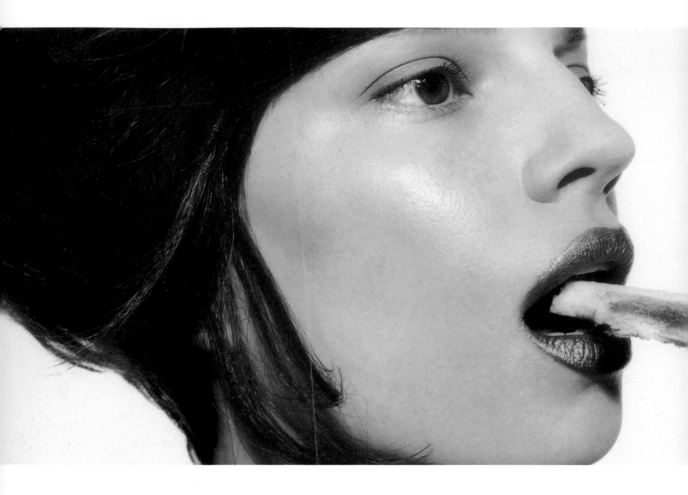

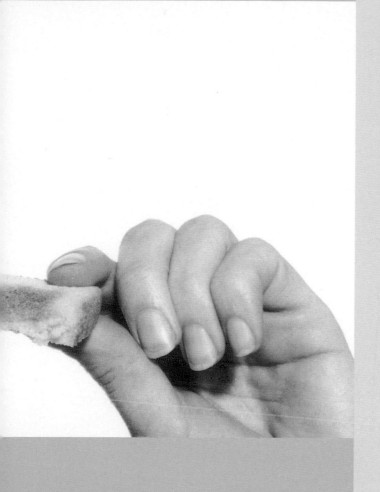

TEXTURE

■ **SHEER** THE MOST NATURAL FINISH. SHEER COATS THE LIPS WITH A HINT OF COLOUR. IT HAS A MOIST FINISH AND ALLOWS THE TEXTURE OF THE LIPS TO SHOW THROUGH.

■ **SHEEN** SLIGHTLY MORE REFLECTIVE THAN SHEER WITH A PEARL ELEMENT IN IT.

■ **SHIMMER** HAS A HIGH CONTENT OF SHIMMER BUT IS NOT FROST. IT HAS A VERY UNIFORMED CREAMY BASE, WHICH ALLOWS THE SHIMMER TO SPREAD EVENLY.

■ **FROST** MUCH MORE SPARKLE THAN SHIMMER AND STANDS OUT MORE. IT MIGHT HAVE LARGER PARTICLES OR JUST MORE PARTICLES OF PEARL IN IT.

■ **CREAM** A MOIST TEXTURE LIKE OLD-FASHIONED LIPSTICK BEFORE THEY GOT CLEVER. REFLECTS LIGHT.

■ **VELVET** RICH AND SMOOTH IN TONE AND QUITE DENSE IN COLOUR. DEMI-MATTE BUT IS NOT POWDERY AND STILL REFLECTS A HINT OF LIGHT.

■ **MATTE** POWDERY AND FLAT. DENSE COLOUR.

■ **GLOSS** LIPSTICK WITH GLOSS. DOES NOT LAST AND HAS A SEE-THROUGH QUALITY. GIVES LOTS OF SHINE.

■ **LACQUER** HIGH GLOSS AND HIGH PIGMENT. ALSO LONGER LASTING AND DENSER COLOUR THANKS TO NEW TECHNOLOGY.

■ **STAIN** ANY COLOUR MADE TO LOOK LIKE IT'S BARELY THERE. ACHIEVED WITH A DAB OF LIPSTICK USING YOUR FINGERS, OR BY USING A PRODUCT THAT IS NOT LIPSTICK SUCH AS CHEEK GEL. GIVES A NATURAL FLUSH WITH NO SHINE.

APPLYING LIP COLOUR

■ LIKE YOUR SKIN, LIPS NEED TO BE IN TOP CONDITION, AND THIS MEANS WELL NOURISHED AND MOISTURIZED. THE SKIN ON YOUR LIPS IS VERY FRAGILE. IT'S LIKE THE SKIN ON YOUR FACE WITHOUT THE TOP LAYER, YET IT'S ALSO THE MOST RESILIENT AND HEALS VERY QUICKLY. BEFORE YOU APPLY ANY PRODUCT, YOU WANT SMOOTH, HEALTHY LIPS. NO DRY SKIN, NO FLAKY BITS, AND NO LEFTOVER MAKE-UP.

■ MILLIE INCLUDES HER LIPS IN HER SKIN CARE REGIME AND NOURISHES THEM WITH HER FACIAL MOISTURIZER TO KEEP THEM SUPPLE AND MOIST.

■ BUT THE LIPS' BEST FRIEND IS LIP BALM. CARRY IT WITH YOU WHEREVER YOU GO AND APPLY WHEN YOUR LIPS FEEL DRY. WHETHER YOU USE A LITTLE GLOSS OR A WHOLE LOT OF COLOUR, IT'S NOT GOING TO WORK IF YOUR LIPS ARE DRY.

■ PICK YOUR TOOLS. ARE YOU JUST GOING FOR A STAIN ON THE LIPS OR SOMETHING MORE INTENSE? DO YOU LIKE TO USE A LIP BRUSH, OR PREFER TO APPLY YOUR LIPSTICK STRAIGHT FROM THE TUBE?

■ LIP BRUSHES ARE A MAKE-UP ARTIST'S ESSENTIAL TOOL, BUT MOST OF US ARE PUT OFF BECAUSE WE HAVE NEVER BEEN TAUGHT HOW TO USE THEM PROPERLY. NOT ONLY CAN YOU FILL IN THE LIPS WITH COLOUR, BUT YOU CAN USE A BRUSH TO LINE THEM INSTEAD OF A LIP PENCIL.

■ THERE ARE TWO MAIN TYPES OF LIP BRUSH: SQUARE AND MOUNTAIN TIP (POINTS INTO A DOME). MILLIE LINES HER LIPS WITH A SQUARE BRUSH AND FILLS THEM IN WITH A MOUNTAIN TIP. THERE IS NO RIGHT OR WRONG WAY, WHATEVER YOU FEEL

COMFORTABLE WITH. BUT EXPERIMENT. JUST REMEMBER THAT YOUR BRUSH SHOULD NOT BE TOO HARD OR TOO SOFT.

■ RUBY SUGGESTS BUYING TWO SETS OF BRUSHES, ONE FOR LIGHTER COLOURS AND ONE FOR DARK. DON'T THINK OF IT AS BEING EXTRAVAGANT, THEY SHOULD LAST YOU A LIFETIME. LOOK AT IT AS AN INVESTMENT.

■ WHEN USING A BRUSH, MAKE SURE YOU PICK UP ENOUGH COLOUR. MOST OF US WIPE IT GENTLY OVER THE COLOUR AND THEN WONDER WHY IT LOOKS SO SUBTLE ONCE ON THE LIPS.

■ DIG THE BRUSH IN AND REALLY MOVE IT AROUND IN THE COLOUR BEFORE YOU APPLY IT, WORKING THE BRUSH BACK AND FORTH.

■ USE THE FLESHY PART OF THE PALM OF YOUR HAND TO TEST THE COLOUR. THE SKIN HERE IS CLOSEST IN TEXTURE TO THAT OF YOUR LIPS. BUT KEEP IN MIND THAT THE COLOUR OF YOUR LIPS IS SLIGHTLY WARMER.

■ RUBY OFTEN USES LIP LINER AFTER SHE'S APPLIED HER LIP COLOUR. SHE PAINTS ON HER LIPSTICK AND GOES OVER THE EDGES WITH A LIP PENCIL. IT GLIDES ON AND BLENDS IN MORE EASILY, AND SOFTENS THE EDGES. USE THIS TECHNIQUE TO ACCENTUATE CERTAIN AREAS OF THE MOUTH, ESPECIALLY IF YOUR LIPS DON'T HAVE MUCH DEFINITION OF THEIR OWN.

■ MILLIE USUALLY PUTS HER LIPSTICK ON FIRST AND THEN REDEFINES HER CUPID'S BOW AND BOTTOM LIP AFTERWARDS BECAUSE SHE LIKES THEM TO STAND OUT MORE. IT MAKES HER LIPS LOOK FULLER.

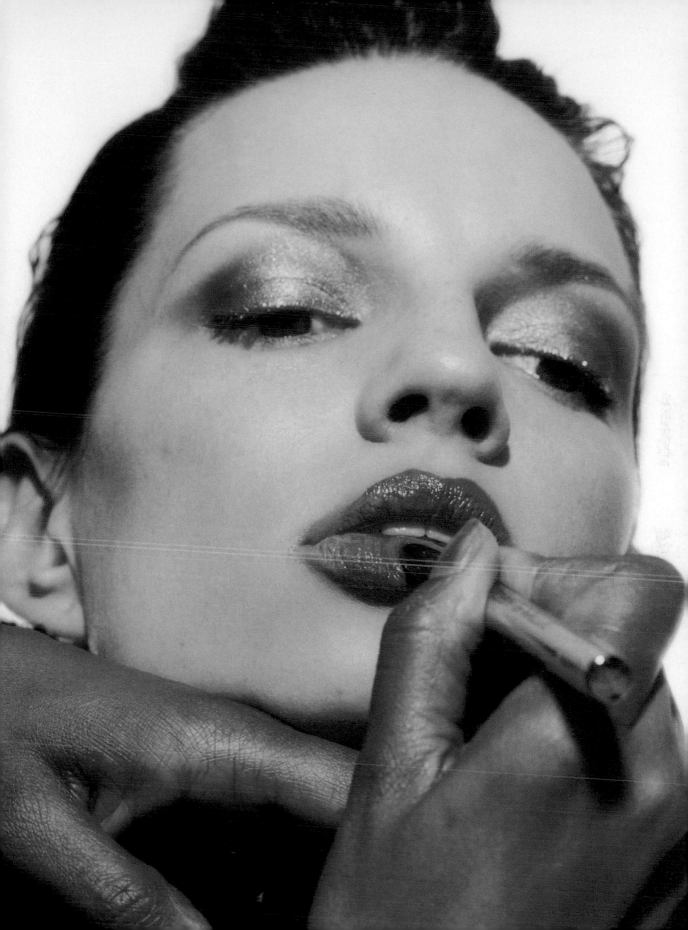

hard

as

nails

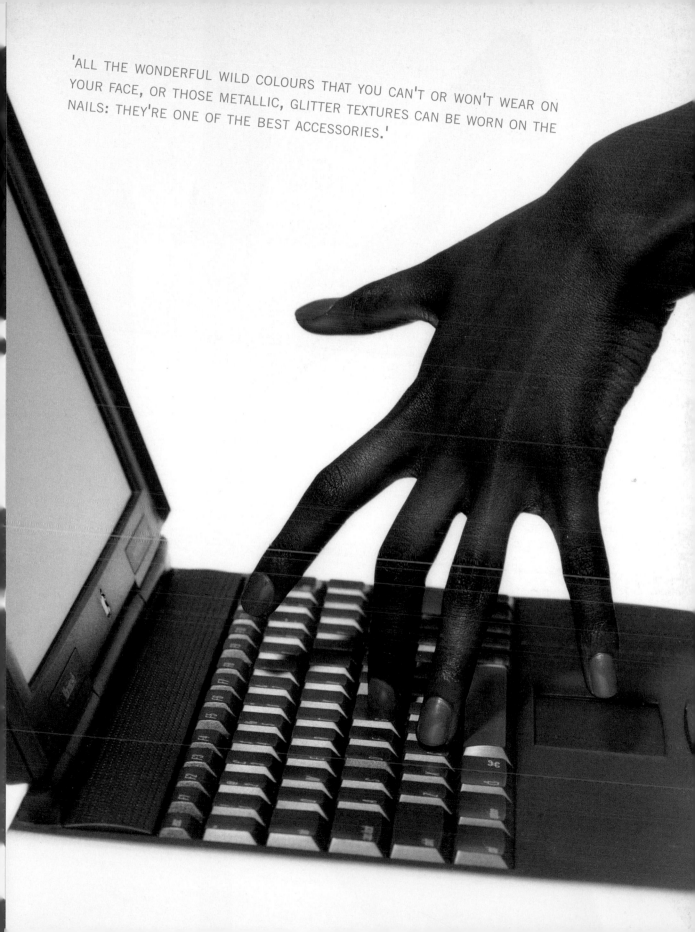

'ALL THE WONDERFUL WILD COLOURS THAT YOU CAN'T OR WON'T WEAR ON YOUR FACE, OR THOSE METALLIC, GLITTER TEXTURES CAN BE WORN ON THE NAILS: THEY'RE ONE OF THE BEST ACCESSORIES.'

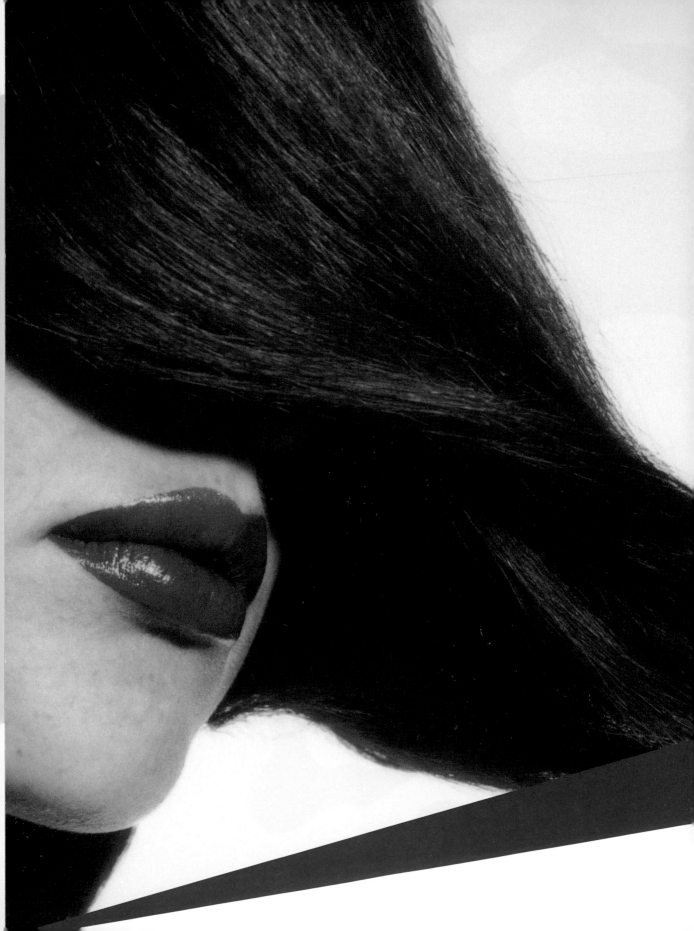

The most important thing about colour is to enjoy it. But it's not about putting all the colours under the sun on your face at one time and hoping for the best. You want to achieve a balance between your eyes, lips and nails to create a beautiful image. Remember that you have many hours, days and weeks to experiment with colour. If you find the most stunning orange eye shadow, why waste it on a face that has orange lips, pink cheeks and loads of mascara? Make the orange eyes the focus for that day.

Too much colour thrown on without much thought also hides what's beautiful about you because you have masked everything that shows your true beauty. Use colour to enhance certain features and make them stand out. You can also use it to downplay other areas. If Millie has spots around her chin she'll wear a dark lipstick – something strong and shocking to detract from

the skin directly around it. It also works the other way round. If you have a feature that you want people to notice, the area around it should be muted. For example, if you have the most beautiful aquamarine eyes and you wear red lipstick, the focus will be on your mouth. A more neutral colour will make the blue stand out.

On the other hand, a monochromatic face, while not drawing attention to any particular area, is still using colour and a statement in itself. But whatever colour you choose, it must not look like an afterthought. If you're going for colour, be bold with it, and make sure it's applied clearly and strongly. And have confidence. Confidence will always be able to carry off colour, and the reverse is true too. If you're shy and uncomfortable wearing it, it won't work for you. Don't think colour is going to make you confident – you need the confidence to wear the colour.

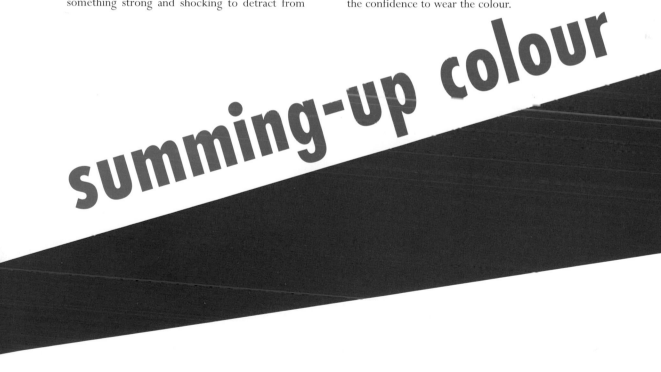

summing-up colour

chapter 6

YOU ALREADY HAVE ONE OF THE ESSENTIAL TOOLS OF THE TRADE – YOUR FINGERS. BUT FOR TRULY BEAUTIFUL MAKE-UP, PROFESSIONAL TOOLS ARE A MUST-HAVE. ONCE YOU KNOW WHAT SPECIFIC BRUSHES DO, THE WORLD OF MAKE-UP IS YOUR OYSTER.

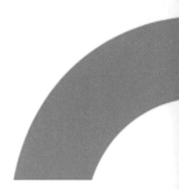

the essentials

the importance of

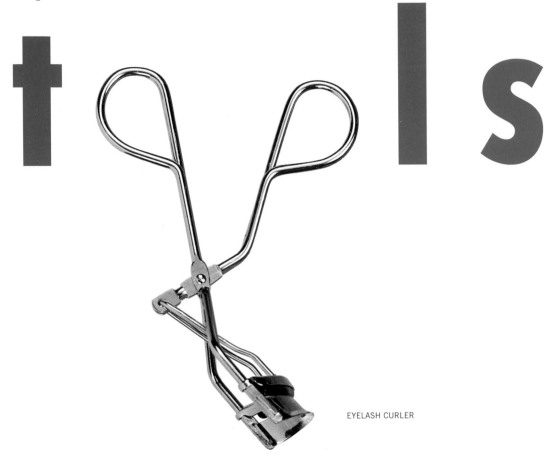

t**oo**ls

EYELASH CURLER

Cosmetics have to be applied with something. You can do a lot of it with your fingers, and it's the preferred method for some people, but it is very rare that from start to finish you can rely on only your fingers. Brushes and tools allow you control and better application to make your make-up look better, last longer and, apart from anything else, be more hygienic.

Buy the best tools you can afford. This does not necessarily mean the most expensive, just the best you can get within your budget.

Nothing baffles Ruby more than a woman who is prepared to spend out on the latest eye shadow palette, yet will be hard pushed to part with money for a brush that will make any eye shadow look better. Think of it as an investment. You don't need hundreds of brushes — many of them can be used for more than one purpose. Just remember that the finer the brush, the more graphic and sharp the effect you're going to get, and the more hair a brush has and the wider it is, the softer the effect is going to be.

choosing the right brushes

A brush has got to feel good. Before you fork out for one, pick it up and feel it. There is nothing worse than a scratchy brush that drags across the skin. There are lots of different hairs to choose from. Goat is the most common but not especially good quality. We are great fans of sable, although synthetic (generally cheaper) are now practically the same in feel and application. We suggest using sable for powder because it distributes better and doesn't stick to the brush, and use synthetic for creams, such as your cream blusher and eye shadow.

Your brushes should be firm so you can draw a line and blend your colour by spreading and smoothing it out. Let the brush do the hard work for you.

clean up

If you look after your tools they will last you for years. And there is no point in having a filthy brush, nothing is worse than using dirty tools. If you let layers and layers of colour build up on a brush, apart from not getting true colour when you apply your make-up, your brushes will lose their shape and therefore their ability to perform their best.

As long as you don't share your brushes, you can get away with cleaning them once a week or fortnight. In an ideal world though, the best way is to clean them after every colour change and in that way your tools are always pristine when you need them. There are brush cleaners out there on the market, but they are specifically designed for make-up artists who clean their brushes constantly, because they dry quickly and the brushes can be used again straight away. However, shampoo or soap will do.

Millie fills the sink with lukewarm water and shampoo, swills the brushes around in the water, rinses them off and lays them on a towel or kitchen roll to dry overnight. Lay the brushes with their tips slightly off the counter top to let the air circulate.

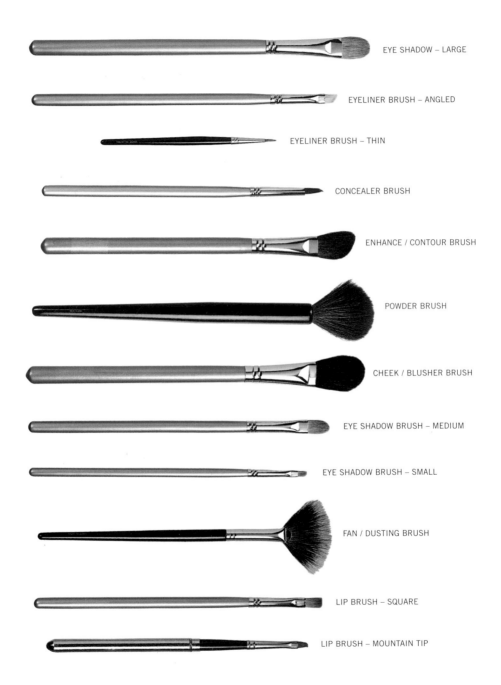

EYE SHADOW – LARGE

EYELINER BRUSH – ANGLED

EYELINER BRUSH – THIN

CONCEALER BRUSH

ENHANCE / CONTOUR BRUSH

POWDER BRUSH

CHEEK / BLUSHER BRUSH

EYE SHADOW BRUSH – MEDIUM

EYE SHADOW BRUSH – SMALL

FAN / DUSTING BRUSH

LIP BRUSH – SQUARE

LIP BRUSH – MOUNTAIN TIP

WHICH BRUSH?

BLUSHER BRUSH: MILLIE PREFERS A TAPERED BRUSH AS OPPOSED TO A FLAT ONE BECAUSE IT BLENDS BETTER. THE HAIR NEEDS TO BE SOFT. KEEP IN MIND THAT IT SHOULD BE SOFTER THAN YOUR POWDER BRUSH BECAUSE IT SHOULD GENTLY CARESS THE CHEEKBONES.

CONCEALER BRUSH: SHOULD BE SYNTHETIC SO THAT IT DOESN'T GET CLOGGED UP. DEPENDING ON THE KIND OF BLEMISH YOU'RE HIDING OR THE AREA YOU'RE TRYING TO COVER, USE IT IN CONJUNCTION WITH YOUR FINGERS. AROUND THE EYES, FINGERS CAN BE EASIER, BUT WITH SPOTS YOU NEED A FINER TOOL. YOU WANT THE BRUSH TO BE ABLE TO COVER AN AREA YET BE PRECISE ENOUGH TO DOT ON A TOUCH OF CONCEALER HERE AND THERE.

CONTOUR BRUSH: AN ANGLED VERSION OF THE BLUSHER BRUSH. BECAUSE YOU'RE APPLYING STROKES OF HIGHLIGHT AND CONTOUR AND BECAUSE IT'S ANGLED, THE LONGER END TRAILS AND SOFTENS THE LINE, SO IT LITERALLY SOFTENS AS IT APPLIES. IT'S ALSO GREAT FOR FOLLOWING THE CURVES ON THE FACE.

EYEBROW BRUSH: GROOMS THE BROWS, REMOVES FLAKY SKIN AND EXCESS PRODUCT, COMBS AND SHAPES THEM INTO PLACE. IT'S ALSO GREAT IF YOU HAVE OVERDONE YOUR EYEBROW SHADOW OR PENCIL BECAUSE YOU CAN USE IT TO BLEND IN THE COLOUR.

EYELINER BRUSH (THIN, ANGLED): WHICH ONE YOU CHOOSE DEPENDS ON WHAT YOU WANT TO ACHIEVE. A THIN BRUSH IS FOR TRADITIONAL LIQUID APPLICATION. YOU CAN ALSO USE IT FOR APPLYING THIN LINES USING EYE SHADOW OR FOR WHEN USING IT WET. AN ANGLED BRUSH IS GOOD FOR POWDER WORK, BUT DON'T USE FOR LIQUID EYELINER BECAUSE IT'S TOO WIDE. THE IDEA OF THIS BRUSH IS TO CREATE A LINE THAT TRAILS AND SOFTENS THE LINE YOU'VE APPLIED, AND ANGLED BRUSHES DO THIS BECAUSE THE LONG END FOLLOWS BEHIND THE SHORT ONE.

EYE SHADOW BRUSH (SMALL, MEDIUM, LARGE): EVERYBODY SHOULD HAVE A MEDIUM EYE SHADOW BRUSH FOR APPLYING COLOUR. YOU SHOULD THEN HAVE A SMALLER ONE FOR MORE FINE WORK AND DEFINING, AND A BIGGER ONE FOR BUFFING AND BLENDING COLOUR.

FAN BRUSH: CAN BE USED INSTEAD OF A POWDER BRUSH. BECAUSE IT REMOVES LESS POWDER IT'S NICE TO USE IF YOU WANT TO LEAVE YOUR FACE LOOKING QUITE MATTE. IT'S ALSO GOOD FOR FLICKING AWAY EYE SHADOW THAT HAS TRICKLED UNDERNEATH THE EYES WHEN APPLYING WITHOUT SMEARING.

LIP BRUSH (SQUARE, MOUNTAIN TIP): BOTH LINES THE LIPS AND APPLIES AND DEFINES THE COLOUR. WHICH ONE YOU CHOOSE IS REALLY DOWN TO PERSONAL PREFERENCE, ALTHOUGH A SQUARE-TIPPED BRUSH IS MUCH EASIER TO LINE THE LIPS WITH. WE SUGGEST YOU KEEP A SQUARE-TIPPED BRUSH AT HOME AND A MOUNTAIN TIP IN YOUR BAG FOR RETOUCHING AND REAPPLYING.

POWDER BRUSH: A POWDER BRUSH IS USED FOR DUSTING OFF EXCESS POWDER, SETTING POWDER, BUFFING UP THE SKIN AND MAKING IT LOOK NATURAL. AS A BUFFER IT SHOULD BE DOMED SO THAT IT ROLLS NICELY OVER THE FACE AND DISPERSES THE POWDER EVENLY.

chapter 7

HAVE A BEAUTY QUESTION? YOU'LL FIND THE ANSWERS HERE.

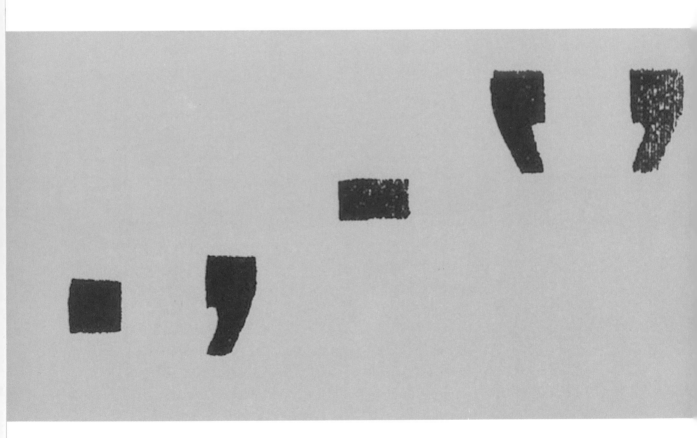

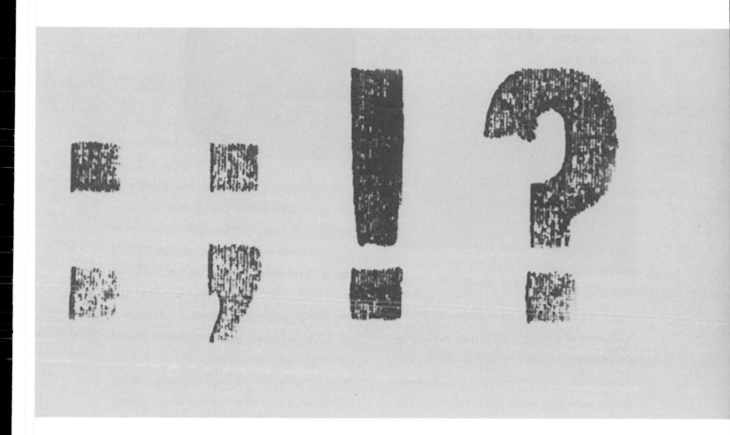

making up

We would also like to thank the following people:

Denise Bates for giving us the opportunity to publish our vision of beauty.

Ciara Lunn for looking after our needs and supporting the project and its tedious details without complaint.

Michael Alcock for making this whole thing happen, and for having the coolest bag in history.

Boots The Chemist for their incredible support to us and Ruby & Millie, and for their investment in our creativity.

Steve Hiett for being a friend and living icon of fashion photography. His support, care and love is undoubtedly the most inspirational aspect of this entire project.

Tamara Sturtz for her direction, determination and dedication to us over the past ten years, and for her impeccable interpretation of our concept. Thank you for putting our vision into words, you did good babe.

Fernando Torrent Visionary of cutting-edge coiffure, he made the images in this book come alive with distinction and direction.

Marcel Bourdon for being the nicest French bloke we've ever met. And for his commitment to making the images within the book superb.

Teresa Nunes for her support of Ruby as assistant make-up artist.

Ivy Thompson for giving us hands and nails to be proud of.

Imogen Fox for getting her hands on brilliant clothes and accessories.

Mike Filby (Tamara's fiancé) for all his love and unfailing patience and support, especially when Tamara was exhausted and pushed to reach her deadline for this book.

Amanda & Peri at Naked for giving us Fernando and supporting us over the years.

Models To all the models who appear in this book we want to thank you for your dynamic personalities and beauty that have made this book prove that as women we can be versatile and independent. Dasha at Premier, Helen Stinton at Premier, Zoe Manzi at Models 1, Annabel Rumble at Select, Susan K at IMG, Madeleine at IMG, Mieko at Assassin, Vanessa Castillejo at Take 2, Clara at Take 2, and Serena at Take 2.

Model agencies To all the agents and bookers that had faith in this project and provided us with top beauties.

Clothes and props Wright & Teague, Nana, MacMillan, Hanro, James Lakeland, Episode, Agnes b, Damart, Boyd, Jigsaw, CK Calvin Klein, Azuni jewellery, The Chair Company, Muji, The White Company.

Spring Studios for a brilliant team who totally looked after us during the making of the images within this book.

Core London Ltd for heroic last-minute digital imaging.

Ruby would also like to acknowledge her mother Rina and her unique family who have not only been there for her with love and support, but who have been the inspiration for much of her life. And to her daughter Reena Hammer who has blossomed into an unbelievable young woman and whose face appears in this book. To all of you, you are something special in my life and your love for me is the most precious thing I have.

Millie would like to thank her partner Steven Severin for his patience and love throughout the past few years and would like to dedicate this book to her daughter Sadie. Your love for me is my reason for living.

to ruby

As a tribute to my partner Ruby who shows me courage, morality and truth, time and time again. I have to thank you for your friendship and partnership through the good times and the bad, the respect I have for you is limitless and your talent, creativity and superb skill as a make-up artist astounds me every time I see you touch a face. I love you truly and will treasure our friendship forever. Love Mill.

to millie

Singularly we have individual talents but together we become formidable. Thank you for bringing and sharing all your unique and unbelievable talents allowing me to benefit from that creative blend and also from your deep and loyal friendship. I look forward to reminiscing with you in our rocking chairs. Amen. Love Ruby.

index